NEW Vegetarian Baby

" Research shows us very clearly that vegetables, grains, beans, and fruits should take center stage. They provide the nutrition children need to grow, and avoid the cholesterol and animal fat that can cause so many problems.

Benjamin Spock, M.D., and Steven Parker, M.D.,
Dr. Spock's Baby and Child Care[1]

Sound vegetarian diets provide a food pattern that is adequate but not excessive in energy, protein, fat, minerals, vitamins, water, and fiber. They meet the needs of the infant or child for growth and development, are age-appropriate, and fulfill any other special health needs that have dietary implications for the individual child.

Pediatric Nutrition Handbook, Fourth Edition[2]

Research shows a carefully planned vegetarian diet can be nutritionally adequate and healthful for children from infants to teenagers.

American Dietetic Association[3]

Well-planned vegan and lacto-ovo vegetarian diets are appropriate for all stages of the life cycle, including pregnancy and lactation. Appropriately planned vegan and lacto-ovo vegetarian diets satisfy nutrient needs of infants, children, and adolescents and promote normal growth.

Virginia Messina, M.P.H., R.D. and Kenneth Burke, Ph.D., R.D.,
*Position of the American Dietetic Association:
Vegetarian Diets*[4]

If foods are chosen wisely, vegetarian diets are healthful. A variety of foods helps ensure an adequate intake of nutrients.

Linda Gay, R.D.,
The Yale Guide to Children's Nutrition[5]

. . . [A] vegetarian diet, with only minor changes in eating habits, can meet all nutritional requirements. This diet has the added benefits of reducing the risk of several degenerative diseases.

Robert Garrison, R.Ph., and Elizabeth Somer, R.D.,
The Nutrition Desk Reference[6]

. . . [A] diet centered on grains, beans, vegetables, and fruits is the natural diet of humans and the one that best supports our optimal health.

Virginia Messina, M.P.H., R.D., and Mark Messina, Ph.D.,
The Vegetarian Way[7]

There are plenty of healthy vegetarian children in the world. Vegetarianism need not be a problem if eating patterns are planned carefully so that benefits of the vegetarian diet are balanced by attention to adequate intakes of energy, protein, calcium, iron, and other nutrients that are less available in plant foods.

Reply to a letter on *NUTRIQUEST*, an on-line service of the
Cornell University Division of Nutritional Sciences[8]

Animal source food is adaptive when there's not enough food, but in a world with abundant and diverse plant foods, animal source food is obsolete and only causes problems.

William Harris, M.D., author of
The Scientific Basis of Vegetarianism[9]

Well-planned vegan diets which include a wide range of plant foods provide all the nutritional requirements of pregnant and nursing women, and their children, from infancy through adolescence. . . . Several studies have shown that vegan women have healthy pregnancies, and that their children thrive. Thousands of healthy children have now been reared on vegan diets, and can expect to look forward to a healthier-than-average adulthood.

Gill Langley, M.A., Ph.D., MIBiol.,
Vegan Nutrition[10]

Vegetarian diets are consistent with the Dietary Guidelines and **”** can meet Recommended Dietary Allowances for nutrients.

Dietary Guidelines for Americans[11]

Also by Sharon K. Yntema

Vegetarian Baby

Vegetarian Children

Vegetarian Pregnancy

Also by Christine H. Beard

Become a Vegetarian in Five Easy Steps!

NEW
Vegetarian Baby

**An entirely new, updated edition
of the classic guide to raising your baby
on the healthiest possible diet**

Sharon K. Yntema

and

Christine H. Beard

MCBOOKS PRESS
Ithaca, New York

Cover photo by Nick Elias.

Library of Congress Cataloging-in-Publication Data

Yntema, Sharon, 1951-
    New vegetarian baby / by Sharon Yntema and Christine Beard.
        p. cm.
    Includes index.
    ISBN 0-935526-63-3 (alk. paper)
    1. Infants--Nutrition. 2. Vegetarian children. 3. Baby foods. I.
Beard, Christine H. II.
    Title.
    RJ216.Y565 1999
    613.2'62'0832--dc21   99-047876

Excerpt page 2 reprinted with the permission of Simon & Shuster, from *Dr. Spock's Baby and Child Care*, Fully Revised and Expanded Edition, by Benjamin Spock, M.D., and Steven J. Parker, M.D. Copyright 1945, 1946, © 1957, 1968, 1976, 1985, 1992 by Benjamin Spock, M.D.; Copyright renewed © 1973, 1974, 1985, 1996 by Benjamin Spock, M.D., Revised and updated material copyright © 1998 by The Benjamin Spock Trust.

Distributed to the book trade by
Login Trade, 1436 West Randolph, Chicago, IL 60607
1-800-626-4330.

Additional copies of this book may be ordered from any bookstore or directly from McBooks Press, 120 West State Street, Ithaca, NY 14850. Please include $3.00 postage and handling with mail orders. New York State residents must add 8% sales tax. All McBooks Press publications can also be ordered by calling toll-free 1-888-BOOKS11 (1-888-266-5711).
Please call to request a free catalog.

Visit the McBooks Press website at http://www.mcbooks.com.

Printed in the United States of America
9 8 7 6 5 4 3 2 1

Disclaimer

The authors and publisher believe that this book outlines an excellent regimen for raising a healthy baby. However, they cannot accept any responsibility for the health of your child should any problems arise. Every child has individual nutritional needs. While using the information in this book, you should consult with your pediatrician, a registered dietitian, a certified nutrition consultant, or a public health nurse about your child's individual requirements.

For Nikolas
—Sharon

For my parents, Robert and Betty Beard
—Christine

The time we take to be thoughtful about how we live is extra time for living better.

Laurel's Kitchen

Contents

About the Authors

SHARON K. YNTEMA was born in Detroit, Michigan in 1951 and grew up on St. Croix in the U. S. Virgin Islands, where her mother first introduced her to a vegetarian diet. She received a B.A. in Psychology from Earlham College and an M.A. in Early Childhood Special Education from George Washington University. Before her son was born in 1978, she worked as a child development specialist at the Day Care and Child Development Council in Ithaca, New York. She still lives in Ithaca where she works as the buyer/bookkeeper for a large independent bookstore. Her vegetarian son continues to be very healthy, smart, and tall, having passed her 5'8" stature by age 14.

CHRISTINE H. BEARD was born and raised in Modesto, California. During her late teens, she studied at the San Francisco Ballet School, and then moved on to earn a B.A. in Mathematics and an M.S. in Physics from San Francisco State University. She became a vegetarian in the summer of 1986 and a vegan in 1989 for ethical reasons, but health concerns soon led her to become interested in vegetarian nutrition as well. After the publication of her first book, Become a Vegetarian in Five Easy Steps!, she received certification as a nutrition educator. In addition to her work with nutrition clients, Ms. Beard writes non-fiction, fiction, and poetry; tutors math; teaches quilting; and participates in various political, community, and activist groups. More information is available at her website, http://www.Life-Dance.com.

Acknowledgments

THANK YOU . . .

to the parents of vegetarian children who shared their experiences with such enthusiasm . . .

to Kris Iwasaki, for sharing her childhood memories.

to the members of the McBooks Press staff for doing such excellent work with such great cheer: Alex Skutt, publisher; Wendy Skinner, editor; S.K. List, copy editor; and Stephen Kimball, marketing director.

to the members of the Sci-Veg Internet discussion group for holding the vegetarian community to a high standard when conducting research and making claims. I appreciate the time many of you took to answer my questions.

to Erik Marcus, for his astute comments which have helped make this a better book.

to my partner, David Goldblatt, for all the usual things.

And last, but not least, to Sharon for allowing me to play with her Baby!

—CHRISTINE

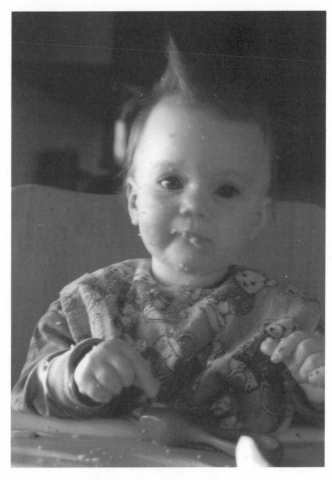

Bella at 14 months, with tofu

Foreword

ONE OF THE greatest gifts you can give your newborn is to raise him or her as a vegetarian. The choice to have a baby is courageous on so many levels—all of which reflect the desire to pass on the gift of life—and what better way to affirm the sacredness of life than to shape your baby's eating patterns in a way that is optimal for health and simultaneously spares other beings from harm?

I often wish I had been raised as a vegetarian, but I also understand my parents' thinking. Back in the 1960s, so little was known about infant and child nutrition that to raise a baby as a vegetarian could get a person criminally charged with child endangerment. Fortunately, the state of nutritional knowledge advanced rapidly during the 1970s, and many assumptions about the food requirements of babies were proven to be untrue. By the early 1980s, it had become clear that a properly planned vegetarian diet is appropriate for people of any age—babies included.

When the first edition of *Vegetarian Baby* was published in 1980, it became an instant classic and, quickly, one of the best-selling vegetarian books in print. Parents around the world have relied on it for reassurance and for making sense of the complex issues that surround infant nutrition. For while nutritionists now agree that vegetarian diets are suitable for babies, it's also clear that there are plenty of ways that parents can go wrong if they lack authoritative information. And just as certain nutritional hazards crop up when you include meat or dairy products in a child's diet, a range of issues must also be considered when you decide to raise your child exclusively as a vegetarian.

Sharon Yntema did a masterful job of researching the dietary needs of vegetarian infants and babies, and the first edition of this book became a bible for a whole generation of parents who wanted something better for their children than a lifetime of fried chicken and burgers. Yet as cutting-edge as this book was when it came out, it must also be said that few books have aged so quickly. For one thing, the state of nutritional knowledge regarding infants has raced ahead during the 1990s, and today we have a far clearer picture of what nutritional issues confront vegetarian babies and how these special requirements can best be addressed. Another factor that prematurely aged the first edition of this book is that it did not specifically address vegan parenting, and during the 1980s and 1990s, growing numbers of parents decided to bring up their children not merely as vegetarians, but as vegans.

For a variety of reasons, many parents are now choosing the vegan path for raising their children. For starters, consider the ethical factors. All animal products—not just meat, but also dairy and eggs—require the killing of animals. As animals age, their milk and egg yields invariably diminish until the time arrives when the animal cannot turn a profit and has to be replaced. As a result, most cows are slaughtered in the U.S. at around the age of five, even though they could live 20 years. Similarly, most egg-laying hens go to slaughter before their second birthday, even though they are capable of living about five years.

So a vegan diet carries some powerful ethical advantages and several health advantages as well. Nutritionally speaking, the closest things you'll find to meat are whole dairy products and eggs. All of these foods are loaded with saturated fat and cholesterol, while they also lack anything in the way of cancer-preventing phytochemicals.

Furthermore, new research has uncovered some dangers in feeding cow's milk to babies and children; potential problems range from obesity to lactose intolerance to intestinal bleeding. With these things in mind, the case for raising your baby as a vegan has never been so strong. But before you resolve to raise your child as a vegan, you'll need to learn about a number of nutritional issues. That's where this book comes in.

For the first time, *New Vegetarian Baby* gives as much attention to vegan parenting as it does to vegetarian parenting. It will give you an overview of eating patterns, risks, and benefits, so that you can decide for yourself where on the omnivore-vegetarian-vegan spectrum you want your family and your baby to be. Whatever choice you make, you'll find the dietary advice you need to help your baby thrive.

Nutritionally speaking, this is an exciting time to be a parent. Never has so much nutritional information been available to parents who want the very best for their children. This book draws much of that information together in an accessible, sensible way to help you guide your baby into a positive relationship with food that will lead to a long and vigorous life. And what greater gift can we give our children?

—ERIK MARCUS, author of
Vegan: The New Ethics of Eating

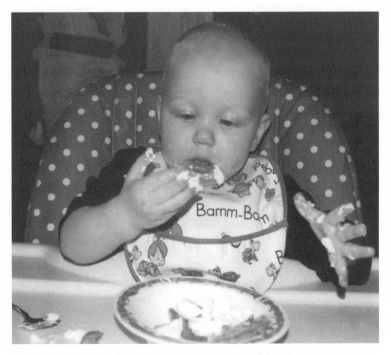

Levi at 17 months, with pumpkin pie

An Idea Whose Time Has Come

IN 1998, in the revised edition of his famous manual on baby and child care, Dr. Benjamin Spock shocked part of the world—and delighted the rest—when he advocated a vegan diet for children. The nutrition section of his book now reads like a vegetarian manual, a far cry from the advice of the 1950s and 1960s when the infamous Four Food Groups— meat, milk, (refined) grains, and (processed) fruits & vegetables—held sway over our nation's eating habits. Given Dr. Spock's reputation as the world's foremost authority on raising children, this is an exciting development indeed, especially for those who have long advocated vegetarian diets.

Sadly, Dr. Spock's death at age 94 occurred shortly before the latest edition of his book appeared, which allowed challenges to his unconventional nutritional advice to pass unanswered by him. His ideas, however, are supported and defended by a growing number of prominent researchers and nutrition experts. And although some authorities persist in the belief that a vegetarian diet is unacceptable for children, a few even equating it with child abuse, their views are challenged by the thousands of healthy vegetarian children—including some who are second, third, and nth generation vegetarians—who have been identified and studied over the past decades.

In other words, not only can children be fed a vegetarian diet from birth, but they can thrive on it, maturing into adults who reach the peak of their genetic potential, with fully realized physical and mental capacities.

The purpose of this book is to offer guidelines which will allow you to raise your child as a vegetarian. By following this sensible advice, you will help your baby to develop healthfully through the first two years of life on a diet that starts with breast milk or formula and segues into a varied vegetarian diet of grains, legumes, vegetables, fruits, nuts, seeds, and perhaps eggs and dairy products.

New Vegetarian Baby retains much of the structure and content of Sharon Yntema's original work, *Vegetarian Baby*, first published in 1980 and revised in 1984 and 1991. Minor alterations have been made to the organization of the book, but the major changes stem from additions and deletions which reflect nearly two decades of nutritional and biological research, information exchanges within the vegetarian community, and cultural and technological advances.

The book begins with a survey of the diets of babies in other cultures, both vegetarian and near-vegetarian, along with a summary of some of the most important research studies performed in the field of vegetarian nutrition. This first chapter is designed to increase your confidence by letting you know you are far from alone in your decision to raise your baby on a plant-based diet. Other parents' successes and errors will also illustrate what works and what does not.

From a cultural and scientific overview, the book moves on to a detailed discussion of the latest knowledge concerning vegetarian nutrition for infants and small children. Nutrition is a complex field but, as this chapter shows, you don't have to be a biologist, medical doctor, or registered dietitian in order to learn to feed your child foods which will amply meet his or her nutritional needs.

You also will learn something about meeting your own nutritional needs. For a vegetarian baby to thrive, the child's parents must be healthy as well, especially the mother, through the months of pregnancy and lactation. The third chapter, therefore, discusses diet from the parent's side. You'll find suggestions on how to manage your responsibilities while providing for your child's needs and how to interact with people who are concerned by your decision to raise your child as a vegetarian. Finally, emotional support is offered in the form of personal interviews with other vegetarian parents.

All children develop at their own pace, but certain basic feeding behaviors and developmental landmarks tend to occur in a specific order within a basic time frame. In the fourth chapter, you will learn what signs to look for so you can offer your baby the right foods in the right way at the right time. Your child will benefit by developing a healthy attitude towards food and mealtimes which will translate into healthy eating patterns later in life.

The next two chapters offer practical information regarding food preparation techniques and feeding guidelines. These chapters are laid out for easy reference so you can find information quickly while juggling a spoon in one hand and a baby in the other!

Frequently asked questions comprise the final chapter. If you have a question not answered in the text, you should find it in this section. If not, resources which you can use to obtain further information are listed throughout the text, in the appendices, and in the bibliography.

One final note: Segments entitled "Sharon's Story" are scattered throughout the book, starting with the following pages. These contain Sharon Yntema's personal observations from the original *Vegetarian Baby*. Although her son is now an adult, her story continues to offer invaluable support and wisdom which you are sure to appreciate as you live with your own vegetarian baby.

SHARON'S STORY: *The Beginning*

When I was approaching adolescence, my mother began to introduce brown rice into our main meals. Soy grits replaced hamburger meat in our spaghetti sauce. Brewer's yeast flavored our orange juice, gagging me, but delighting my baby brother who knew no different. We still ate meat, but meatless meals appeared more often. Walnut Acres sent us shipments of "health foods" that weren't available where we lived. I remember the excitement when one of these packages would arrive, filled with interesting foods I still did not recognize.

During the time I was in college, vegetarianism grew in popularity. It had the aura of an esoteric secret being revealed. To most of us, it meant adding brown rice and sprouts and homemade bread to our diets and removing meat. I ate with friends off campus who were vegetarians and I enjoyed those meals much more than I did the standard college fare. I knew the difference well because I worked in the school cafeteria, serving meat meals, but leaving as soon as my shift was over to eat my vegetarian meal. I lived with meat-eaters during my last two years in college and had to pay only a small portion of the weekly budget since meat comprised the major cost of meals. This economic advantage continued after college. I lived in cooperatives for several years, and I believe I paid about a third the amount paid by the meat-eaters.

It wasn't until I was pregnant that I began to realize how little I really knew about vegetarian nutrition. Despite this lack of knowledge, I was healthy, partly because my mother had ingrained in me some healthy eating patterns from such an early age.

My husband has been a much stricter vegetarian than I for many years. While I eat dairy products and, occasionally, seafood, he prefers to eat few dairy products and eggs, and no meat. While I was pregnant, we decided that we wanted to raise our baby as a vegetarian, and to learn enough about nutrition so that we would know what we were doing. We knew that raising a child as a vegetarian was not a venture anyone should undertake in ignorance.

As I studied vegetarian nutrition, I found that the specific needs of babies were often ignored in books, or, at best, mentioned only briefly. There was no one book that answered all my questions. This omission nagged me as I proceeded to raise my vegetarian baby.

However, I became knowledgeable in a number of necessary areas through extensive reading and wanted to share my information with other parents. I was invited to give a workshop on the subject of feeding babies meatless meals. The response from this workshop and from informal conversations with other parents confirmed my conclusion that there was a need for a handbook on vegetarian nutrition and cooking for babies.

I hope that this book as a whole will free vegetarian parents from any hesitations created by the meat-eating culture surrounding us. All new parents experience fears that they may not be doing the best for their children, whether it be in the area of discipline, education, or feeding. Many parents simply do not trust themselves to know intuitively what is best. This attitude is not odd in a culture such as ours which separates families and encourages the nuclear family to solve all its problems alone. Our culture offers very little support for new parents, providing no replacement for the wisdom of grandparents and others in an extended family. Often, no grandparents are nearby to offer advice, and even if there are, many new parents feel that advice from another generation is an intrusion.

Most children who grow up eating meat do so because their parents simply passed on the meat-eating habit they themselves inherited. New vegetarians don't have inherited traditions to give their children; they must create their own. A new vegetarian is like an adult learning a second language. Children can speak their native language with ease and fluency by the time they are five years old; they have grown up hearing and speaking nothing else. An adult doesn't have as easy a time. However, the adult novice can bring to the situation a tool that children don't yet command: analytical reasoning. The adult can look at some examples, formulate a rule, and consciously apply that rule to new situations. The results may be halting speech for a while, but as the adult practices speaking and listens to others talk, fluency increases. People who learn vegetarianism as a "second language" must use the same kind of analysis, experimentation, and practice if they are to become nutritionally "fluent." Their children, however, can then grow up as "native" vegetarians.

Vegetarian parents need to become nutritionally "fluent." They need to know they can raise their children with the same principles they live by without endangering their children's health. This reassurance can come through talking with other people who have raised healthy vegetarian children, obtaining nutritional information which specifically addresses their needs, and learning from other cultures. The greatest reassurance will be watching our children grow to be healthy adults who can practice vegetarianism with "native" ease.

Vegetarian Babies in Science and Society

Nature's methods, perfected over millions of centuries, are always purposeful and nearly always right.

> Dr. Jelliffe, under the auspices of
> the World Health Organization[1]

One day in the future, everyone will be as aware of the harmfulness of eating animal products as we today are aware of the necessity of physicians' washing their hands before delivering a baby.

> Harvey Diamond[2]

SHARON'S STORY: *Exploring Other Cultures*

The first reading I did was an exploration of other vegetarian cultures, searching for clues as to what those people fed their babies and why. This reading also gave me confidence that our decision to raise our baby as a vegetarian was the wisest one.

Being a vegetarian is more than not eating meat. Finding out about other peoples whose whole lives are based on vegetarian philosophy can be deeply inspiring. Every group of vegetarians has some ideas that will aid in our growth as vegetarian parents.

Having a feeling for the universality of vegetarianism, whether as an integral part of a culture or as a solution to the problems of malnutrition, can help new vegetarians to better understand their own philosophies.

• • •

MANY SOCIETIES and cultural groups around the world have either greatly reduced or completely excluded meat, and sometimes other animal products, from their diet for religious, philosophic, and economic reasons. The majority of Indian yogic groups, for example, are vegetarian because their members do not want to take the life of another living being. Similarly, some Christian orders, sects, and organizations believe that the Bible and other religious writings specifically speak against the eating of flesh. Among them are the Seventh Day Adventists, approximately half of whom are vegetarian for both religious and health reasons.

This chapter describes various cultures which have successfully incorporated either a plant-based or a completely vegetarian diet as a way of life, whether on the basis of philosophy or economy, or both. These cultures offer a wealth of knowledge regarding infant-rearing practices, food preparation, and other issues of interest to members of the modern vegetarian movement. Data are scant in some cases and profoundly detailed in others, but taken together they are a testament to the ability of humans of all ages to thrive under a wide variety of conditions while eating vegetarian foods.

No such presentation would be complete without mention of some vegetarian cultures which have experienced health problems, usually due to premature weaning, poor hygiene, or restrictions among plant foods, in the course of their elimination of animal products. These isolated cases are equally instructive as they show what practices to avoid when raising your vegetarian baby. The goal of these investigations is the growth of a new vegetarian culture that incorporates the best of other such cultures while rejecting those elements that have been shown to be harmful. Your vegetarian baby will reap the benefits of this knowledge.

What Kind of Vegetarian Is Your Baby?

The definition of the word "vegetarian" has become rather fluid over the years, so any book on the subject needs to define its terms.

Vegetarian
Vegetarians do not eat meat or meat by-products of any kind. All vegetarians, therefore, eschew red meats, poultry, fish, seafood, gelatin, lard, animal-based broth, and similar foods.

Lacto-Ovo Vegetarian
"Lacto" refers to milk and other dairy products, while "ovo" (or, more properly, "ova") refers to eggs and egg products. Some people are either lacto-vegetarians or ovo-vegetarians, but most include both eggs and dairy products in their otherwise non-meat diet. The American Academy of Pediatrics (AAP), the National Academy of Sciences (NAS), the American Medical Association (AMA), and the United States government are among the many respected institutions which have sanctioned the lacto-ovo vegetarian diet.

Vegan
Vegans eat no meat, meat by-products, dairy products, or eggs. Some people prefer to use the term "strict vegetarian" to distinguish such dietary vegans from ethical vegans who also avoid eating other animal products, such as honey, and seek cruelty-free clothing, household products, cosmetics, medicines, and entertainment.

Although many doctors and nutritionists still lack basic knowledge of what constitutes a healthy vegan diet, the American Academy of Pediatrics, the American Dietetic Association, and the Institute of Food Technologists are three major organizations which state that a carefully planned vegan diet can be adequate for infants and small children.[3]

Veg*n
A comprehensive term, mostly used on the Internet, which includes both lacto-ovo vegetarians and vegans.

Pisco-Pollarian

Many people who consider themselves to be vegetarian actually are pisco-pollarians, meaning they avoid mammalian ("red") meats but still eat poultry ("pollo") and fish ("pisco") or other seafoods. In common parlance, they often are referred to as near-vegetarians, semi-vegetarians, or partial vegetarians. If meat constitutes only a small part of the diet, it can more accurately be called a plant-based diet. This diet is increasingly being adopted by those meat-eaters who are concerned with their health, and it is well accepted by the medical and nutrition communities, but it should not be confused with a truly vegetarian diet.

Macrobiotic

Macrobiotics is a dietary philosophy, rather than a diet, which is based upon the Eastern concept of yin-yang and which emphasizes eating locally grown, seasonal foods. A macrobiotic diet is not necessarily vegetarian, but many vegetarians eat a macrobiotic-style diet. While the macrobiotic philosophy has much to recommend it, some macrobiotic practices are potentially harmful for young children, and those will be specifically pointed out in the section on macrobiotics so parents can avoid associated problems.

Fruitarian

Fruitarians eat only plant foods that can be obtained without ultimate harm to the plant, but exactly what that includes is very much up to the individual. A fruitarian diet that includes both raw and cooked nuts, seeds, grains, legumes, fruits, and some fruit-type and leafy vegetables, is essentially a vegan diet as explained above, but it still will lack certain important plant foods such as root vegetables. A fruitarian diet generally is not, therefore, adequate for a child, and even more restrictive fruitarian diets which consist only of raw fruits and seeds are not recommended as a steady diet for anyone, either adult or child, because the variety of foods is too limited for long-term health.

Raw Foodist

Since our more distant ancestors, like all animals, had access only to raw foods, some people consider it unnatural to eat anything else. Raw foods diets usually are plant-based but may contain raw honey, raw eggs, raw dairy products, and raw meats, depending on individual philosophy. A completely raw foods diet can be very risky for babies as it is difficult for them to obtain enough calories and other nutrients, and it may expose them to harmful organisms, especially if raw animal foods are used (with the exception, of course, of breast milk). Raw plant foods are an important part of a healthy diet, however, and recipes based on raw plant foods can be included in the diets of toddlers and older children.

An interesting conclusion can be drawn from the above definitions, namely that essentially all babies are lacto-vegetarian, or even vegan, until seven or eight months of age! That is a natural result of feeding them breast milk or formula during infancy and weaning them onto cereals, fruits, and vegetables. Only when concentrated protein foods are introduced in the latter part of the first year is there a divergence between the diets of vegetarian and omnivorous children. But since legumes, whole grains, nuts, and seeds are part of a healthy diet for vegetarians and omnivores alike, even then the difference is not great among nutritionally aware families.

The Farm

Vegetarian parents sometimes feel alone in their efforts to raise vegetarian—and especially vegan—children. A success story, therefore, is quite encouraging. The Farm, a spiritual community founded in Tennessee in 1971, is an example of a vegetarian culture that works. A vegan diet was the standard on The Farm until 1983 when The Farm ceased being a strictly communal organization, and some members resumed eating eggs and dairy products.[4]

Over the decades, The Farm has been home to many individuals and families. The population peaked in 1982 with around

750 adults and an equal number of children.[5] Approximately two hundred people still live on The Farm today where they continue to practice "simple living and self-reliance" as well as conducting businesses like Mushroompeople and the Book Publishing Company.[6]

A landmark dietary study was conducted at The Farm by researchers from the Centers for Disease Control in Atlanta, Georgia. In 1984, the researchers directly gathered height and weight data for 144 children living on The Farm. That data was supplemented with growth measurements and demographic information previously gathered by The Farm's own health clinic and ETHOS, a Farm research organization. The final analysis included data for 404 children for the years 1980 to 1984. The ages of the children ranged from four months to ten years, and the majority had been vegan for the first two years of life (not counting breast milk).

The final report appeared in the September 1989 issue of *Pediatrics*. The researchers found that the children were growing normally, at rates generally falling within the 25th to 75th percentiles. As a group, the children's growth tended to be very slightly below the median for the general population: mean heights were 0.2 to 0.7 cm shorter and mean weights 0.1 to 1.1 kg lighter than the national averages for different age groups.[7] The researchers concluded that ". . . the growth of The Farm children even though modestly less than that of the reference population, showed no evidence of marked abnormality. [With] attention to weaning foods and nutrient intake, a group of children raised with a relatively strict vegetarian diet (vegan) can achieve adequate growth."[8]

The New Farm Vegetarian Cookbook describes in detail how vegan children on the Farm are fed. No animal products, including milk and eggs, are used in the traditional Farm diet. Soy milk manufactured on The Farm is fortified with vitamins A, B-12, and D, and supplementation of vitamin B-12 is obtained through the use of fortified nutritional yeast.

Mothers are encouraged to nurse for at least six to eight months. Strained vegetables, fruits, and soft, bland processed cereals are introduced to babies after four to six months, and starches and unprocessed grains after six to eight months. Soy milk, soy yogurt, and tofu are introduced when the baby is seven to eight months old, but not before, because his or her digestive system is not ready for soy products until that time.

Soups made from legumes other than soybeans (e.g., well-blended and diluted split pea soup), and well-mashed, de-skinned beans, are given to Farm children a month or so after soy products. Whole soybeans are hard to digest unless they are very well cooked; some children can't eat them until age two or three years.

Parents at The Farm have community support in their efforts to raise healthy vegetarian children. The Farm exemplifies a vegetarian culture based on knowledge of nutrition, cultural borrowing, and group sharing. Because Farm children have been objectively found to be healthy, The Farm diet model is an excellent one for other vegetarian parents to follow.

RESOURCES

The New Farm Vegetarian Cookbook edited by Louise Hagler and Dorothy R. Bates (Book Publishing Company, 1988).

Voices from the Farm: Adventures in Community Living edited by Rupert Fike (Book Publishing Company, 1998). http://www.thefarm.org

Seventh Day Adventist

Physicians are not employed to prescribe a flesh diet for patients, for it is this kind of diet that has made them sick. Seek the Lord. When you find Him, you will be meek and lowly of heart. Individually, you will not subsist upon the flesh of dead animals, neither will you put one morsel in the mouths of your children.

Ellen G. White[9]

Another successful vegetarian community is that of the Seventh Day Adventists, a significant number of whom are lacto-ovo vegetarians and some of whom are vegan. The unique character of this Christian religion largely derives from Ellen G. White

(1827–1915), who is seen by the church to be a prophet and whose writings "are considered to be an authoritative source of truth."[10] According to the Ellen G. White Estate, those writings include more than 5,000 periodical articles and 49 books, as well as many manuscripts. Her writings on nutrition are largely responsible for the vegetarian nature of the Seventh Day Adventist church, and her work in establishing schools and hospitals can be seen in the many Seventh Day Adventist institutions that exist today, including Loma Linda University in California where "research and education in vegetarian nutrition have been a focus . . . for 75 years."[11]

One such research study followed over 27,000 vegetarian and omnivorous Seventh Day Adventists in California for a period of 21 years and established that "those consuming predominantly vegetarian diets had lower age-specific mortality rates than did non-vegetarians, even after controlling for factors such as history of smoking or chronic disease."[12]

Another study looked at Canadian Seventh Day Adventist women who were long-term vegetarians and found that their iron and zinc status "appeared adequate despite their low intake of readily absorbed iron and zinc from flesh foods and their high intake of total dietary fiber and phytate."[13] The results of this study underscore our limited knowledge of how food constituents react inside the body as opposed to in test tubes and theoretical models, and it offers pregnant and nursing vegetarian women some reassurance of their ability to absorb adequate iron and zinc from their foods, even when some of those foods contain mineral-binding substances such as phytates.

Researchers have also studied Seventh Day Adventist children. For example, a study comparing Seventh Day Adventist children with non-Adventist, Caucasian children in Southern California found that "vegetarian children and adolescents on a balanced diet grow at least as tall as children who consume meat."[14] Another report reviewed several growth studies and concluded that while "11- to 12-year-old girls following a lacto-ovo vegetarian diet are 3 to 3.5 cm shorter than omnivore girls of the same age," this difference "is most likely due to a delayed onset of the pubertal growth spurt" and that "this maturation delay may carry potential health benefits in adult life."[15]

The combined result of these and other studies has been the almost total acceptance of lacto-ovo vegetarian diets by the nutrition community.[16-21] The Seventh Day Adventist model thus is an excellent one for lacto-ovo vegetarians to follow. As stated in another review of data from Seventh Day Adventists: "An early establishment of a healthy lifestyle seems to be of decisive importance in the risk of later disease."[22]

RESOURCES

Ten Talents by Frank J. Hurd and Rosalie Hurd (The College Press, 1985).

Total Health and Food Power: Principles of Healthful Living and Outstanding Vegetarian Recipes from Glendale Adventist Medical Center by Rose Budd Ludlow (Woodbridge Press, 1986).

Vegetarian Nutrition and Health Letter
School of Public Health, Loma Linda University
1711 Nichol Hall, Loma Linda, CA 92350
(888) 558-8703; http://www.llu.edu/llu/vegetarian

Ellen G. White Estate Branch Office
Andrews University
Berrien Springs, Michigan 49104
(616) 471-3209; http://www.egwestate.andrews.edu

Macrobiotics

Above all, learn from your children. Observe them carefully— they will teach you to have confidence in life. . . .

George Ohsawa, founder of the modern
macrobiotic movement[23]

The macrobiotic (literally "great life") philosophy, which originated in ancient Japan, is based on a concept that divides the aspects of the universe into two polarities, yin and yang. Basically, yin is the quiet principle: simplicity and receptiveness; yang is the moving principle: effortless and creative action. According to this philosophy, a balance between the two opposites is necessary for optimal spiritual, mental, and physical development. Foods are classified according to the yin and yang they contain, and recipes balance combinations of foods.

George Ohsawa, the author of *Zen Macrobiotics*, the major work designed to explain macrobiotics to the Western world, stressed again and again that "macrobiotic living is not a rigid adherence to a set of rules."[24] He suggested that parents should study the philosophy of macrobiotics and increase understanding of themselves before having children. He believes that parents should be aware that children have good intuition about eating and drinking. For example, Ohsawa advised parents to trust that a child knows when he or she is thirsty, and to provide liquids accordingly.

The issue of milk use is important in macrobiotic theory on infant nutrition. In a chapter on dairy products in his book, *Basics and Benefits of Macrobiotics,* Edward Esko states that the "expansive" nature of milk makes it an ideal food for the rapidly growing baby, but that after weaning, drinking milk is ". . . harmful both physically and spiritually."[25] Macrobiotic practitioners do recognize the importance of having abundant calcium levels, but they maintain, as do other authorities, that it is possible to obtain sufficient calcium from vegetable origins rather than from dairy products. From birth to about six months of age, the macrobiotic child nurses, gaining sufficient calcium from mother's milk. The child is then weaned over the course of the following 12 to 14 months. High-calcium foods, such as leafy green vegetables (especially kale, mustard greens, collards, and dandelion greens), sea vegetables, nuts seeds, and soy milk are emphasized.[26]

Blackstrap molasses, soybeans, carob, and fruits (especially dried fruits like figs, apricots, and dates) also supply calcium.

Emphasizing the ability to get sufficient calcium from plant sources alone, Ohsawa and his followers also believe that it is wrong to drink milk from other animals. They feel that the milk of an animal is intended only for its offspring and is not suitable for feeding to other species. Since eggs also are not a traditional part of the macrobiotic diet, most vegetarian macrobiotic diets tend to be vegan. The standard vegetarian macrobiotic diet for people living in temperate climates consists largely of cooked foods from the following groups:

Whole grain cereals (50 percent)
Vegetables (20 to 30 percent)
Beans and sea vegetables (5 to 10 percent)
Soups (5 to 10 percent)
Seasonal fruits (occasional)
Nuts, seeds, and other natural snacks (occasional)

Even though milk from other animals is unacceptable in the macrobiotic diet, all mothers are encouraged to nurse their children until at least one year of age. If a macrobiotic mother's milk supply is low during this time, she is encouraged to eat a sweet brown rice gruel covered with tahini or ground walnut sauce. Ohsawa suggests adding grains and cereals in puréed form to the nursing baby's diet at about six months of age.

Many studies of vegetarians are actually studies of people practicing macrobiotics, some of whom follow a true vegetarian diet, and some who include small amounts of meat (usually seafoods) in their diets.[27-34] And while many principles of macrobiotics can be beneficial—the emphasis on organically grown, whole foods, for example, and the attention given to being fully aware of one's food, chewing thoroughly, and not eating heavily right before sleep—certain other practices are potentially harmful, and it behooves all vegetarian parents to be aware of them. Details on some of the following items will be given in later chapters, but a general list of macrobiotic child care practices to moderate or avoid are as follows:

1. Restricting salt. In the macrobiotic philosophy, salt is seen as a very potent food additive which should be restricted in the diets of young children, but zealous restriction of your

child's sodium intake is not necessarily a good idea. Infants naturally prefer bland foods, but some salt, preferable iodized, can be an important part of a toddler's diet, and adult-style restrictions should wait until the child is older. (*See Sodium, page 83.*)

2. **Delaying the introduction of vegetables.** George Ohsawa recommended that children not eat vegetables until one year of age, but this practice can deprive a baby of important nutrients like iron and calcium just when they are most needed. Macrobiotic parents should note that Michio and Aveline Kushi, perhaps the foremost students of Ohsawa, recommend feeding vegetables soon after beginning a child on cereal grains.[35]

3. **Avoiding certain classes of plant foods.** The macrobiotic proscription against entire types of foods such as "nightshade" vegetables and tropical fruits can restrict a vegetarian diet so much that health becomes hard to achieve, especially for small children who already tend to be picky eaters.

4. **Avoiding all or most raw foods.** A combination of raw and cooked foods will result in the best nutrition.

5. **Relying completely on local, seasonal foods.** While local produce grown in its traditional season can be fresher, more interesting, and better for the environment, it also can lead to poor nutrition if the local soils have an imbalance of certain elements or the variety is overly limited. The inclusion of foods from other places can improve the quality of the diet, especially during winter months.

6. **Using homemade milk substitutes for infants.** If a baby cannot be breast-fed for some reason, a commercial infant formula is the only responsible alternative. Milks made from nuts, seeds, grains, and soybeans can be excellent additions to the diet of older children and adults, but they are no substitute for breast milk or commercial formula during the first two years of life.

7. **Eschewing the use of supplements and fortified foods for

both mother and child. Ideally, food will supply all nutrient needs, but sometimes supplements are essential to ensure good health. One of the most important examples is the macrobiotic reliance on sea vegetables, spirulina, tempeh, and other such foods to obtain vitamin B-12. As will be discussed in detail later, these foods are not reliable sources of true B-12 (cyanocobalamin), and supplements must be used when there are few or no animal products in the diet. (*See vitamin B-12, page 77.*)

8. **The use of too many high-fiber foods while using too few high-fat foods,** which can lead to failure to thrive due to poor nutrient absorption and too few calories.

9. **Depending on superficial indicators** such as thumb-sucking, cranial shape, eye size, hair whorl direction, and the like, to determine nutritional requirements and development, as is suggested in Michio and Aveline Kushi's first child care book, *Macrobiotic Pregnancy and Care of the Newborn.* While children are individuals and do have different abilities and needs, there are much better ways to assess them.

10. **Relying on food and home remedies to cure a child of serious illnesses** like pneumonia and meningitis, rather than seeking out standard medical care (again suggested in the Kushis' first book). Western medicine certainly is not perfect and has much to learn from alternative therapies, including dietary and herbal therapies, but there are times when natural remedies alone are not enough. As the authors of one study on religion-motivated medical neglect state: "Applied to minor or self-limited problems, many non-medical practices are probably benign, but may lead to avoidable morbidity and mortality with more serious ailments."[36] Your child depends on you to exercise good judgment as to when home care is enough and when a doctor is called for. Fortunately, the Kushis have moderated their stance in their more recent book, *Raising Healthy Kids.* Their first book cannot be recommended.

Raising Healthy Kids by Michio Kushi and Aveline Kushi with Edward Esko and Wendy Esko (Avery Publishing Group, 1994).

The Kushi Institute
Box 7
Becket, MA 01223
(413) 623-5741; http://www.macrobiotics.org/Ki.html

Vega Study Center
1511 Robinson Street
Oroville, CA 95965
1-800-818-8342; http://www.vega.macrobiotic.net

Macrobiotics Online (the Kushi Institute and One Peaceful World) http://www.macrobiotics.org

Chinese

Buddha first taught himself to avoid the sin of killing any living creature; he wished that all people might know the blessedness of a long life.

The Teaching of Buddha [37]

An enormous health and nutrition research effort was undertaken in China and Taiwan during the 1980s, with numerous analyses published in articles and books in the years since then. The formal name of this study is the China-Cornell-Oxford Project on Nutrition, Health, and Environment, but it is more popularly known as the China Project or the China Study. The goal of the study was to investigate the relationship between diet and disease, especially the degenerative diseases, such as cancer, which plague industrialized nations. China was chosen because previous data indicated that cancer rates varied widely between differing regions. Since the living habits of the populace were fairly stable within each region, but varied among regions, the survey yielded a wealth of information regarding the influence of diet on health. The China Study is of great interest to vegetarians because the results strongly suggest that a plant-based diet is the healthiest type of diet, especially when followed over one's entire life.

Data were obtained in 1983–84 from 6,500 men and women from 65 Chinese counties. A second survey in 1989–90 included the people originally studied and added another 20 counties from both China and Taiwan for a total of 10,200 adults. The researchers gathered information through a questionnaire, three-day diet histories, food samples, and medical examinations. Data on 1973–75 mortality rates from various diseases were recorded during the first survey, while data on 1986–88 mortality rates were added to the second.

The following is a summary of the results as reported on the Cornell University website. The data is attributed to the numerous publications which have resulted from this study.

1. On average, the total protein intake of the Chinese was 65 percent of the average United States intake, with between zero to 20 percent of that protein provided by animal-based foods, compared to 60 to 80 percent in the U.S.

2. People eating more plant protein tended to grow to a greater height than those eating smaller amounts of plant protein. This suggests it is the amount of protein, rather than its source, which most affects growth.

3. The study yielded evidence that adding even small amounts of animal foods, and specifically animal protein, to an otherwise all plant diet elevated total and LDL cholesterol levels. Blood cholesterol levels in China averaged 127 milligrams/dl with a range of 90 to 170, compared with the United States average of 212 and range of 170 to 290. Triglyceride levels also were lower (97 milligrams/dl in China versus 120 milligrams/dl in the U.S.).

4. The Chinese eat substantially less fat than do people in the United States. During the first survey (1983), the average fat intake was 14 percent of calories in China versus 36 percent in the U.S. At the time of the second survey (1989), those numbers had changed to 19 percent and 34 percent,

respectively. Not surprisingly, the Chinese are significantly thinner than Americans, with an average Body Mass Index of 20.5 versus the Americans' 25.8. Interestingly, the calorie intake of the Chinese was 30 percent higher than that of people in the United States.

5. The Chinese diet contains three times the U.S. fiber intake—33.3 grams versus 11.1 grams per day—mostly from cereal grains.

6. The study participants were found to have healthy iron levels when eating high-fiber diets even though fiber is thought to reduce iron absorption.

7. The researchers found a much lower incidence of osteoporosis in China even though calcium intakes were quite low according to U.S. standards, averaging 544 milligrams per day. There was some evidence that dairy products might increase bone density, but that increase did not appear to result in further reduction of osteoporosis. The lower protein intake (*see above*) is thought to be a protective factor, as is the less sedentary Chinese lifestyle.

8. A much lower incidence of breast cancer was found in rural China, and breast cancer risk was linked to fat consumption and high levels of estrogen and testosterone in women. Bowel cancers also were much less prevalent in China than the United States, perhaps due to the much higher fiber content of the Chinese diet.

9. On the other hand, the Chinese were found to have a much greater incidence of stomach cancer, theoretically due to overuse of fermented and salty foods which can reduce the acidity of the stomach and allow infection with *Heliocobacter pylori,* an organism that has been linked to damage of the stomach lining. Liver cancer rates also are very high in China because of the high rate of hepatitis infection.

10. High blood levels of the anti-oxidants beta carotene and vitamin C, which are found in plant foods, were associated with lower death rates from many cancers.

The overall conclusion of the study is that "a substantial change in American dietary patterns from animal-based foods to plant-based foods must occur for there to be a substantial change in disease incidence patterns."[38] Furthermore, a paper by the leader of the project, T. Colin Campbell, states that "there appears to be no threshold of plant-food enrichment or minimization of fat intake beyond which further disease prevention does not occur."[39] In other words, if people in the United States want to reduce significantly their risk of developing degenerative illnesses such as heart disease and many types of cancer, they need to reduce their intake of fat and animal protein substantially while, at the same time, increasing their intake of fiber through the use of whole foods (but not too many fermented and high-salt ones). A whole foods vegetarian diet is an obvious choice.

RESOURCES

China Project
http://www.human.cornell.edu/dns/chinaproject/chinaproject.
html
Diet, Life-style, and Mortality in China: A Study of the Characteristics of 65 Chinese Counties by J. Chen, T.C. Campbell, J. Li, R. Peto. (Oxford University Press, Cornell University Press, and People's Medical Publishing House, 1991).

East Indian

He who injures harmless beings from a wish to give himself pleasure, never finds happiness, neither living nor dead. . . . He who permits the slaughter of an animal, he who kills it, he who cuts it up, he who buys or sells meat, he who cooks it, he who serves it up, and he who eats it, are all slayers.

The Laws of Manu V, Hindu text [40]

Harmlessness is the only religion.   Jain maxim [41]

Another major culture with a strong vegetarian tradition is that of the Hindus and Jains of India. For the most part, Hindus eat a lacto-vegetarian diet while many Jains strive to follow an ethical vegan path. Since vegetarian foods have been eaten in India for many generations, the cuisine is highly developed and has greatly influenced the cooking of Western vegetarians.

Indian cooking relies heavily on rice and potatoes; flat breads made of wheat, lentil, or chickpea flour; lentils and chickpeas; dried fruits and chutneys; sesame seeds and tahini; coconut; vegetable oils; and a large variety of vegetables, herbs, and spices. Milk products are used in sauces, yogurts, and cooling drinks such as riata, as well as the clarified butter product called ghee. Fresh fruits turn up too, but generally in small amounts.[42]

Because of their tendency to favor vegetarian diets, Hindus have been the focus of many nutrition studies, not only in India, but also in other countries with large Indian populations, such as Great Britain. The results of the studies vary, as might be expected from a large population of people on so many different educational and socioeconomic levels.

One researcher found that, while vegetarian infants in India can experience retarded growth, probably due to "poverty [and] intestinal infestation" which affects the quality and quantity of food as well as absorption of nutrients, "when people of Indian origin migrate to developed countries and maintain their vegetarian dietary practices but consume more dairy products, the impact of the vegetarian diet on growth is more limited." The same researcher also notes that vegetarian Hindu women experience somewhat shorter pregnancies (by four to five days) and their babies tend to be slightly lighter (190 to 240 grams), possibly due to too few calories coupled with low intake of certain nutrients such as iron, folate, and vitamin B-12.[43-44]

On the other hand, a study of the growth of children in South India found that for children older than three years, both height and weight growth rates were significantly higher for piscarian children than for omnivorous ones. The researcher hypothesized that one possible reason for the difference was sanitation—in a place with little or no refrigeration, plant foods and fresh fish are less likely to cause illness than is red meat.[45] (The researcher for this study defined the participants as vegetarians but noted that all of them ate fish. They were, therefore, actually piscarians.) Taken together, these articles make it clear just how important it is for children and pregnant women to have access to a good variety of plentiful, clean food.

As in macrobiotics, food is often used medicinally in India through the ancient practice of Ayurveda, which literally means "the science of life." According to author and physician Rudolph Ballentine, the "science of nutrition in Ayurveda is vast and comprehensive and is not separated from pharmacology. Since no distinction is admitted between foods and drugs, herbal and mineral substances that are used in the preparation of food are thought to be equally important medicinally as those that are given separately."[46] There is a germ of truth in this in that the foods we choose can affect our health, especially in the long term. However, claims that specific foods and herbs have miraculous healing powers are more questionable. Spice your family's foods for flavor rather then for medicinal purposes, unless the benefit of some particular item has been supported in reputable studies. Even then, dietary and herbal remedies should not take the place of standard medical care, but should only be used in conjunction with it.

Japanese

The vegetarian cuisine of Japan has been greatly influenced by Buddhism. Not all Buddhists are vegetarian, but some, such as the Tibetan Buddhists and Zen Buddhists, have practiced vegetarianism for many generations and have developed exquisite culinary traditions as a result. These traditions have permeated many Asian cultures, which in turn have had a great impact upon the health of native regional peoples as well as giving the world such wonderful foods as tofu, tempeh, and seitan. As one Japanese Zen Buddhist abbess observes:

> There are two main reasons why shojin [temple] cooking is based on vegetables and sea plants. The first relates to the geography and topography of the Japanese islands and

the second to the Buddhist religion. Generally, it is easier to grow vegetables in Japan than to raise animals on a paying basis. . . . To this fact was added the dictates of the Buddhist religion [which] sets forth five proscriptions [including] "thou shalt not kill" [which] applies not only to human beings, but to cattle and swine as well as to birds and even insects.[47]

The traditional Japanese diet is based on rice, although other grains (millet, barley) and starchy vegetables (taro, sweet potatoes) also are used. The rice generally is accompanied by vegetables, including sea vegetables, and some legumes, especially tofu and other soy products. Fruit is a small part of the diet, most often in the form of the umboshi plum, although melons and other fruits certainly are much prized. The main animal foods for omnivorous Japanese are seafoods, with small amounts of poultry and other meats. The connection to the macrobiotic diet is obvious.

Over the past century, and especially since the end of World War II, the Japanese diet has undergone enormous changes, with a large increase in the amount of meat, fat, and processed Western-style foods. This is perhaps most marked in the urban areas.[48] The result is a sort of "natural laboratory" with a homogenous population where some people eat the traditional plant-based diet, some eat Westernized fare, and yet others were raised on the former before switching to the latter as adults. Japanese who have emigrated to other countries also have been studied extensively.

One outcome of these studies has been a greater understanding of the role certain foods play in the cause and prevention of diseases such as breast cancer and heart disease. For example, one study found that a diet high in soy foods was associated with lower cholesterol levels for both men and women, and another uncovered some evidence that soymilk can reduce serum estrogen levels in women.[49-50] Green tea also appears to have cancer prevention benefits.[51-52] The high level of sodium in the Japanese diet does appear, however, to be associated with a higher incidence of stomach cancer, just as it was in the China Study.[53]

Although most studies concentrate on adults, the diet of Japanese children is also of interest to researchers, especially since it has changed drastically in recent decades. As an example, over seven million Tokyo schoolchildren were tested for non-insulin dependent (Type II) diabetes over the two decades between 1974 and 1994. The researchers found that the rate of this type of diabetes has continued to increase since 1976, and they theorize that the increase stems from a combination of less exercise and more animal fat and animal protein.[54]

To get some idea of how much the Japanese diet has changed since World War II, consider the following recollections of a middle-aged Japanese-American woman who spent the first four years of her life in Japan.[55] The diet she remembers eating as a child was plant-based and largely made up of traditional foods with a few exceptions. Notable was the use of white rice and whole plant foods (vegetables, legumes, fruits) as well as the small amount of animal foods (mostly seafood) and refined sweets. A pre-war Japanese diet probably would have been similar save for the pastries and dairy products.

Breakfast was typically a half-croissant filled with chocolate, or a brioche stuffed either with custard or the more traditional sweet adzuki-bean paste (*an* or *anko*).

For lunch, the pre-school children usually had a *bento-baco* (lunch-box) brought from home and arranged with great care— white rice in the center, often with an umeboshi plum in the middle, with a corner arrangement of sweet, shredded shrimp and either a toasted nori sheet or a sprinkle of *furikake* (literally "sprinkles," it is a mixture of seaweed, rice crackers, sesame seeds, and bonito shavings).

Snacktime in the afternoon consisted of cows' milk or miso soup. The cows' milk at home was thick and creamy, probably raw. Her grandfather roasted sweet potatoes in a large charcoal grill to sell out his door, a common practice at that time, and sometimes well-caramelized sweet potatoes were served as a snack or a dessert.

Dinner had two basic variations. The first was similar to lunch but with more variety—a small portion of fish, miso soup, rice, and assorted pickled vegetables such as a Napa-type cabbage.

Tofu was cubed and served with *shoyu* (soy sauce), grated daikon, and bonito flakes. The other dinner was rice with a stew (*ni-mono*—literally "stewed things") of daikon, potato, and carrots into which was placed bean thread cake (*konnyaku*) and fish cakes. The fish cakes were prepared in such a way that they had widely differing textures, colors, and shapes, even though the taste was uniform.

Very few desserts were eaten. Sometimes there were the caramelized sweet potatoes. Occasionally, there was fruit, such as tangerines, and during the winter, roasted chestnuts. The most memorable dessert accompanied storytellers who sold homemade, unwrapped sugar candies as well as a clear, taffy-like substance made from millet which was twirled onto a pair of chopsticks. But the woman remembers her parents becoming angry when she ate such refined sweets.

RESOURCES

Zen Vegetarian Cooking by Soei Yoneda with Koei Hoshino (Kodansha International, 1982).

Pacific Islanders

The culture of small islands, especially tropical and sub-tropical ones, meant the people there traditionally ate plant-based diets because their islands were too limited in area, with too few animal species to afford meat-eating on a regular basis, with the notable exception of fish and other seafoods (and sometimes cannibalism!). While not vegetarian, such piscarian-oriented diets offer insight into human nutrition and the feeding of babies and children on a plant-based diet.

Hawaiians

. . . [T]he native Hawaiian people, once known to be tall, slim, athletic and healthy, today have among the poorest health in the nation.

Terry Shintani, MD, JD, MPH[56]

Dr. Terry Shintani is the Director of Preventive Medicine at the Waianae Coast Comprehensive Health Center and a clinical faculty member of the University of Hawaii School of Medicine and School of Public Health. In 1989, he founded a program known as the Waianae Diet. His goal was to reverse the extremely ill health experienced by many people of native Hawaiian descent. At present, these people suffer an unusually high rate of degenerative diseases such as obesity and diabetes, but that was not always the case. Photographs and descriptions from early European explorers and colonizers of the Hawaiian Islands paint a picture of robust, healthy families much different from what is observed today.[57]

The Waianae Diet is based on the traditional diet eaten by the native Hawaiian people, an eating pattern very similar to the traditional Japanese diet described above. The main starch is taro (often made into poi) which is accompanied by plentiful fruits such as bananas and papayas, along with green vegetables, sea vegetables, and small amounts of fish and poultry. During the program, the participants experienced significant improvement in their weight, cholesterol, and blood pressure readings, as was reported in the *American Journal of Clinical Nutrition* and the *Hawaii Medical Journal*.[58-59]

A similar program called the Hawaii Diet has since been developed for the general population. In 1997, a three-week trial of the Hawaii Diet resulted in similar health improvements for the 23 participants, including the governor of Hawaii. Examples include an average weight loss of 10.8 pounds, average cholesterol decrease from 205 to 157, average triglyceride decrease from 238 to 152, average blood pressure decrease from 130/79 to 120/75, and great improvement in blood sugar readings for those with diabetes.[60]

Although these studies were of adults, extrapolation from these and other studies strongly suggests the study participants would not have developed such health problems in the first place had they eaten a whole foods, plant-based diet for their entire lives.

Waianae Book on Hawaiian Health by Terry Shintani (Waianae Coast Comprehensive Health, 1990).

Dr. Shintani's Hawaii Diet by Terry T. Shintani (Pocket Books, 1999).

Dr. Shintani's website http://hfma.hisurf.com/shintani

Marquesans

A [breadfruit] tree was planted for each newborn child and henceforth the fruit of that tree belonged to the individual.[61]

The Marquesans live on the Marquesas Islands in the South Pacific, a part of French Polynesia. They occupied the islands some 2,000 years ago and, like other Pacific islanders, were "discovered" by European explorers, most notably Captain James Cook in 1774, four years before his arrival in Hawaii.[62] The islands are very rugged and lie in the tropic zone, with warm weather all year round. Traditionally, the villages have been built near once-volcanic mountains. In general, volcanic soil is rich in minerals, resulting in excellent nutrient quality of crops grown on it.

When Europeans came to the Marquesas, they brought diseases and customs which had a devastating effect on the islanders. The late 18th-century population of approximately 100,000 had dropped to around 1,200 by 1923. But during the intervening decades since, the population has slowly increased to over 7,000.

In a book called *The Appetites of Man*, authors Sally De Vore and Thelma White reported that Marquesan babies were raised on vegetarian diets and only introduced to seafoods when they entered adulthood. While that claim is questionable, the following description of Marquesan baby food is probably reasonably accurate: "After a year or so of breast-feeding, the mother supplements the infant diet with a sort of porridge made from the albumen of the immature coconut and starch from grated native arrowroot. A nutritionist who visited the islands analyzed the chemical composition of the coconut through its various stages of development and discovered that the very young nut is low in calories which increase as the coconut matures. They are extremely rich in phosphorus, iron, thiamin, riboflavin, niacin, ascorbic acid, and vitamin E, and when eaten in combination with breadfruit, taro root, or other starchy vegetables, provide the major portion of nutrients needed for good health."[63]

This description is not meant to be taken as a recommendation of how to feed a baby, as the diet described is much too limited in scope for good health. Instead, it is included as an interesting example of the type of starch-based fare which traditionally has been used in many cultures and which forms the basis for today's healthy vegetarian diets.

Babies in Non-Industrialized Countries

More than half the young children who die in developing countries are malnourished. This does not mean that they starve to death but that poor nutrition lowers their resistance to killer diseases. It is at the stage when the human body is developing that malnutrition has its most severe effects. . . . Four main types of malnutrition are the most damaging. Protein-energy malnutrition . . . iron deficiency . . . iodine deficiency . . . [and] vitamin A deficiency.

World Health Organization[64]

Malnutrition is a very common problem in many non-industrialized countries. Often, animals are few in number, and usually the meat that is available is so high-priced as to be unaffordable to most families. Added to these factors is the influx of highly processed foods from industrialized nations which destroys any naturally healthy diet patterns these peoples might have had in the past.

Malnutrition is so common in some countries that several international efforts have been made over the last century to solve the problem. The World Health Organization, the Indian Council of Medical Research, and the Medical Research Council in London are among the many groups working against malnutrition. Their basic philosophy is counter to the traditional U.S.

assistance approach, and was described by D. B. Jelliffe, a former World Health Organization Visiting Professor of Pediatrics: "The spread of technological civilization has so far done little to help [malnutrition] and in many cases may have worsened the position by destroying or making impossible old and well-tried beliefs and practices without supplying the means for newer methods."[65]

Jelliffe's suggested solution to malnutrition may seem too vague and vast, difficult to grasp for people who've become used to depending on modern technology: "No absolute rules for infant feeding can be laid down and methods must be varied to suit the particular locality. . . . intended improvements must always be based on . . . local customs and beliefs."[66]

After a preliminary assessment of the nutritional status of infants in 14 subtropic and tropic countries, Jelliffe developed a wide range of recommendations to improve infant feeding practices. Although he encouraged the use of animal foods wherever possible, he acknowledged that animal products were widely unavailable in those countries, and said, "It is of great importance to make the best possible use of all locally available plant protein foods."[67]

He then looked at the various cultures to determine what locally available plant protein foods might best be used. In Egypt, he considered a mixture called *mhallabiah* to be "the most suitable local food for the weanling." Mhallabiah is a mixture of cornstarch, ground unpolished rice, ground almonds, milk, sugar and water. In Calcutta, a gruel made of boiled germinated grams (legumes) was considered of greatest nutritional significance, since an increase in the content of ascorbic acid, carotene, niacin, thiamin, riboflavin, and protein is produced by the process of germination. In Lebanon and Syria, burghul (a wheat preparation) and hummus (a chickpea preparation) are cited as two important foods. In Damascus, the two are mixed together, two parts burghul to one part hummus, and a little sour milk is added to make a smooth, appetizing paste.

Another food, *kishkeh,* is made "by adding 3.5 litres of leban (soured milk) to 2.5 kilograms of burghul. After drying, the final product is reported to keep for at least a year."[68] In Bengal, a combination of various legumes and rice was already being used by adults; a paste could be made to adapt this mixture for the young child. In Turks Island, a dish of boiled, sieved red peas, and rice could be similarly used. In Indonesia, a steamed rice and tofu dish was considered to be of high value.

Dr. Jelliffe considered legumes to be "undoubtedly the most valuable vegetable food."[69] Chickpeas (garbanzo beans) are in turn the best legume; a palatable paste is most easily made from them. Jelliffe reported that chickpeas prepared with wheat, bananas, and palm sugar were used successfully in infant feedings in the eastern Mediterranean area.

One of the highest priorities in the improvement of infant feeding recommended by Jelliffe was better maternal nutrition, with breast milk as the only infant food for the first six months of life and as a major food for as long as possible thereafter. Good maternal nutrition, he argued, prevents many problems caused by unsanitary food preparation and storage, as well as by the lack of money to buy more expensive baby food products. When considering what the best weaning foods are, he commented: "All over the world, in the temperate zone as well as in the tropics, the first semi-solid foods are almost always starchy gruels and pastes. . . . there is no reason to believe that this is not the correct method of initiating this phase of infant feeding although . . . this must be rapidly followed by a much wider range of foods, including particularly plant proteins."[70] Finally, Jelliffe put considerable emphasis upon working with the various cultures to develop a sense of community spirit and pride within town and village areas in order to effect long-term improvements in infant nutrition.

In 1974, the Working Party of the Indian Council of Medical Research reported on their studies of weaning and supplementary foods in six areas of India. *Kwashiorkor*, a protein-calorie deficiency disease, was highly prevalent in all areas in young children. They stated that "protein-calorie malnutrition is essentially a disease that occurs during the crucial transitional phase of a child's life from breast milk to other types of foods."[71]

In order to combat this problem, the Working Party developed many recipes made almost entirely of plant proteins. The criteria for the recipes were:

1. they are based on "foodstuffs available locally, and . . . traditionally acceptable to the community. They do not contain any processed ingredient or food material which has to be brought from the outside."[72]
2. they must be preparations capable of easily being cooked at home;
3. they must be able to be made at home in bulk and stored for some time;
4. once in storage they must be easily available to be used as "instant" infant food by mixing with water or milk.

An additional criterion was that the foods be highly acceptable to the children was a criterion, because it was felt necessary for them to consume the foods in amounts which provided 300 calories and 6 to 8 grams of protein, in addition to their usual diets, to combat kwashiorkor. Here are some of the recipes developed by the Working Party of the Indian Council of Medical Research.

Khicheri
75 grams rice
100 grams spinach
50 grams lentils
10 grams oil
Proteins: 19.3 grams,
Calories: 549

Khichuri
50 grams rice
60 grams potato
15 grams oil
50 grams lentils
60 grams papaya
Proteins: 17 grams,
Calories: 554

Foxgram porridge
30 grams sprouted foxgram flour
(local legume)
10 grams roasted groundnut flour
25 grams ripe plantain
(variety of banana)
Proteins: 11 grams, Calories: 217

Cholam adai
25 grams cholam flour
8 grams groundnut oil
20 grams roasted Bengal gram
(chickpea) flour
4 teaspoons water
18 grams jaggery (palm sugar)
5 grams coconut scrapings
Proteins: 7.4 grams, Calories: 325

The recipes were tested on 200 children between the ages of six months and three years. All showed significant growth in weight and height over a 12-month period. Also, hemoglobin levels taken from children receiving these recipes showed significant increases. The one problem with the studies was that nutrients such as vitamins A and B-complex were not considered in the development of recipes since the aim was primarily to combat kwashiorkor. Although these recipes do contain some of the necessary vitamins and minerals because they include whole food ingredients, isolating only a part of the nutrient needs of a child is not the best way to produce healthy people. In the conclusion of this study, the Working Party stated: "It is generally agreed that the problem of protein-calorie malnutrition can only be solved by educating rural communities to effectively utilize inexpensive locally available foods . . ."[73]

Although it is not explicitly stated, the indirect message from this research is that a plant-based diet is generally the most economical, practical, and acceptable path to follow in combating malnutrition in young children in non-industrialized nations. And although the research cited above was conducted some time ago, the same type of "Food mixes . . . containing the staple cereal of a country and additional ingredients that complement cereal proteins, such as nuts and seeds" continue to be used to similar effect.[74-76]

Other Studies of Vegetarian Children

Many studies of the nutritional status of vegetarian children have been conducted. Often, however, the results of particular studies, and especially negative ones, are generalized to reflect on the health of all vegetarian children, which is a very inaccurate and irresponsible practice on the part of scientists, medical professionals, and journalists. This situation has somewhat improved over the past decade, but it still behooves vegetarian parents to be knowledgeable about both major and minor studies in order to learn what practices work and which do not, and to be able to respond to the generalizations of others. Several important studies already have been discussed in the above sections, and a few others are briefly described below. More examples, as well as a discussion of how to evaluate research studies, are included in Sharon Yntema's book, *Vegetarian Children.*

Black Hebrews

And God said, Behold, I have given you every herb bearing seed, which is upon the face of all the earth, and every tree, in which is the fruit of a tree yielding seed; to you it shall be for meat.

Genesis 1:29,30

According to an article in *Society,* "the Black Hebrews believe that the Middle East was once part of African culture and the Jews [who] were dispersed by the Romans traveled as far as West Africa. Black Hebrews from the U.S. settled in Israel beginning in 1967 and live simply, eating a vegetarian diet and wearing only natural fibers."[77]

The Black Hebrews are a small community of strict vegetarians who experienced a tragic level of malnutrition among their infants as was reported in an article which appeared in the October 1982 issue of *Pediatrics.* The babies were exclusively breast-fed until three months of age, and the breast milk was found to be deficient in carbohydrate, protein, and fat, most likely because of the poor diet of the mothers. The weaning diet was limited—"fruits, vegetables (with a wide variation depending on seasonal availability), oats, yeast, and almond or 'soya' milk."[78] The soy milk was a dilute homemade preparation and was "the single most important constituent of the infants' diet between 3 months and 1 year of age." As a result, a large number of the infants "showed evidence of protein-calorie malnutrition, iron and vitamin B-12-deficient anemia, rickets, zinc deficiency, and multiple recurrent infections." Other children showed signs of growth retardation starting with the introduction of weaning. Eight of the children had died at the time of the report.

This study underlines the importance of learning and applying the principles of good nutrition. Pregnant and nursing mothers must be well fed; infants require adequate breast-milk or infant formula for many months; and the weaning diet must consist of a good variety of highly nutritious and calorie-dense foods so as to support normal growth.

Additional Case Studies

Many Rastafarians eat a restricted vegan diet without supplementation, and a few case studies have reported problems with malnutrition in Rastafarian infants. According to a 1988 review of vegetarian children, "Four Rastafarian infants in England were found to have nutritional rickets after having been weaned. . . . Another 12-month-old Rastafarian infant had vitamin B-12 deficiency, possibly because of low B-12 concentration in the mother's breast milk, perhaps a reflection of the mother's own marginal B-12 stores."[79]

More recently, two babies of strict vegetarian mothers developed symptoms of severe vitamin B-12 deficiency due to lack of sufficient vitamin B-12 in their mother's breast milk. One of the children developed normally to age nine months at which point deficiency symptoms appeared. The other began having problems at seven months. Fortunately, vitamin B-12 therapy rectified the problem in time so the damage was not permanent.[80]

Case studies are, by their very nature, limited in scope and so should not be extrapolated to the vegetarian community as a whole, but such isolated incidents are instructive because they make it clear just how important a varied diet and sensible supplementation can be for an infant. As more vegan foods are fortified with vitamin B-12, and other nutrients such as vitamin D, the rare cases of dietary deficiency may well become a thing of the past for vegetarians just as they have in the general population.

Contrast those studies with a longitudinal study of British vegan children born to vegan parents which was conducted starting in

1968. The number of children studied was small, but more were added as time went on. All the children were breast-fed for at least six months, and most for well over a year. The weaning diet consisted of grains (especially whole grain bread), legumes, nuts, fruits, and vegetables. Soy milk and nut milks were used as were between-meal snacks of bread, biscuits, fruits, and nuts. Few refined sweets were given to the children, but dried fruit and molasses were used. Some parents gave their children vitamin D supplements; most also made sure their children were exposed to sunlight. Almost all the parents also gave their children vitamin B-12 supplements or fortified foods.

The result? "The average nutrient density . . . of the vegan diets were [sic] higher for most nutrients with the exceptions of Ca [calcium] and fat compared with the average UK diet." Furthermore, "Heights, weights, and head and chest circumference measurements were inside the normal range for the majority of children . . . although there is a tendency for vegan children to be smaller in stature and lighter in weight than non-vegetarian children."[81] The size difference was theorized by the researchers to be due to low fat intake coupled with overly large quantities of fruits and vegetables, which resulted in a lower energy intake. Other than that, this diet is similar to the successful Farm diet described earlier which confirms it as a good model, so long as some higher energy foods are added to increase the energy intake.

Long-term Health

When a child is malnourished, it's usually because the parent is unaware of the nutritional information necessary for good health, and since we live in a non-vegetarian culture this is perhaps more likely to happen with vegetarian children than omnivorous ones. If a parent, or even a group of parents, is trying something that is not accepted by the mainstream culture, their attempt is tremendously hindered. That is why it is vital for vegetarian parents to read books such as this one, to obtain the information that is not readily available elsewhere.

The disastrous mistakes made by the Black Hebrew community are a prime example of how not to feed your own vegetarian baby. Fortunately, since the time of that report, many more studies of vegetarian children have been conducted, and it has been established that vegan children can grow normally if fed a calorie-sufficient, well-balanced diet.

Reports of research that focus on the positive results of raising children on a plant-based or vegetarian diet are much more useful than media scare stories. Researchers do vegetarians a favor when they focus upon how parents feed their healthy vegetarian children, as do the scientists at Loma Linda University. Such research is still in its infancy, however, so not much is known about how a vegetarian diet in childhood will affect long-term health. Studies on adult vegetarians suggest that they share many health benefits, some because of diet, and others due to various lifestyle practices common to vegetarians such as exercising, and avoiding tobacco and alcohol. Chances are your vegetarian baby will have:

1. less likelihood of becoming obese;

2. a lower risk of lung cancer and alcoholism;

3. less risk of developing hypertension, coronary artery disease, non-insulin-dependent (type II) diabetes, and gallstones;

4. and possibly a lower risk of developing breast and colon cancer, diverticulosis, kidney stones, and osteoporosis.[82-84]

T W O

The Healthy Vegetarian Baby

Life is life's greatest gift. Guard the life of another creature as you would your own because it is your own.

Lloyd Biggle, Jr.[1]

 A HEALTHY BABY comes from healthy, nutritionally aware parents. Because a baby, both before and after birth, is developing more quickly than at any other time of life, he or she has different nutritional needs than an adult. Being aware of these needs, and knowing how to satisfy them, is the way to have a healthy child, whether vegetarian or omnivorous.

The reason most meat-eating families in our society manage to provide the nutrients a child needs, without much effort or nutritional study, is that animal foods are readily available and meat does contain substantial protein, B-vitamins, trace minerals, and other important nutrients. On the other hand, diets which contain a large proportion of animal products and refined foods can be low in nutrients such as folate, carotenes, and vitamin C that are abundant in whole plant foods. Animal products also have a number of unwanted properties such as high levels of cholesterol and saturated fat; lack of fiber; potential contaminants such as pesticide residues, hormones, and food-poisoning organisms; and a high cost of production—economically, environmentally, ethically, and spiritually.[2-6]

The goal of this chapter is to provide the basic nutritional information you need to supply your baby with a diet which contains all the necessary nutrients for normal growth while avoiding the problems associated with eating animal products. If you already are a vegetarian, many of these facts will be familiar but, as you read, keep in mind that being a vegetarian parent is slightly different from being a vegetarian. The difference lies in the responsibility you have towards another being who is completely dependent upon your care. By learning as much as you can about vegetarian nutrition for babies, you will be better equipped to supply your child with appropriate nutrients for healthy growth.

Please keep in mind that even though a chapter on health and nutrition must necessarily include specific information on nutrient allowances and the reasons why we need sufficient amounts of each nutrient, health is more than the sum of these nutrients. Health also includes the love that surrounds a child, and his or her general emotional and intellectual well-being, in addition to the physical condition that can be more easily measured. Vegetarian parents must remember to include in their baby's diet iron, calcium, zinc, and vitamin B-12, but they also should always remember that diet is just one part of raising a healthy vegetarian baby.

What Is "Health"?

Health is not easy to measure. The word often refers only to bodily health, to that state in which all bodily systems are functioning efficiently, but even this definition is not always clear cut. Peggy Pipes, in her college textbook, *Nutrition in Infancy and Childhood*, offers the following definition: "A normal healthy child grows at a genetically predetermined rate that can be compromised or accelerated by undernutrition, imbalanced nutrient intake, or overnutrition. Progress in physical health is one of the criteria used to assess the nutritional status of populations and of individuals."[7]

This definition is useful because it gives a clear picture of some of the difficulties inherent in judging a child's growth. For example, how can anyone ever know what the predetermined genetic rate of development is for any one child? The criterion "progress in physical health" has often been interpreted to mean "bigger is better," which unfortunately has led to much childhood obesity and premature sexual development.

The best definition of health takes into consideration each child's unique needs, family history, and developmental patterns. Does the child seem happy? What is the rate of weight gain? How big are the parents and other closely related family members? What illnesses has the child had? What is the child's normal energy level? A doctor tries to compile all of this information when examining a baby.

When discussing nutrition with your pediatrician, be aware that all doctors will carry their own dietary biases into the appointment. A physician who believes that vegetarian babies are less likely to be healthy than meat-eating ones may worry about the baby's welfare. A worried doctor can foster worry in a parent, and a worried parent may create tension in the child about eating. If a doctor thinks all children should triple their weight by a certain age, and should be eating cereals by the age of three months, or thinks all babies need iron supplements by the age of four months, then these beliefs will influence the way the doctor sees the child and interacts with the parent. Guidelines can be difficult to use as they were intended; sometimes they become absolute rules.

Good health, then, can be viewed only subjectively, and so must be determined by a combination of objective knowledge, experience, and intuition. A health professional who has had few vegetarian patients may tend to rely less on experience and more on the available data about the optimal amounts of vitamins, minerals, carbohydrates, proteins, and fats on which babies seem to thrive. When discussing your baby's diet with a pediatrician, remember that dietary data, objective though it may be, must be interpreted correctly. Recommendations are developed for populations, not individuals, and your baby's needs may be different (either higher or lower) than the standard. The members of the

National Academy of Sciences, who develop the official nutrition tables for the United States, explain:

> Diets are more than combinations of nutrients . . . present knowledge of nutritional needs is incomplete. . . . RDA should not be confused with requirements. . . . Differences in the nutrient requirements of individuals that derive from differences in their genetic makeup are ordinarily unknown. Therefore, as there is no way of predicting whose needs are high and whose are low, RDA (except for energy) are estimated to exceed the requirements of most individuals and thereby ensure that the needs of nearly all are met.[8]

That statement is not very helpful if you want to know exactly how much iron or calcium your child needs. But if you understand that the guidelines are only guidelines, and adapt them to your individual child, the result should be a healthy baby. Regular checkups at the pediatrician's office will offer reassurance and allow the doctor to notice any changes you, in your day-to-day handling of the baby, may not. A doctor who is knowledgeable about vegetarian nutrition certainly is preferable, but any competent doctor can provide the input you need to monitor your child's growth and overall health status, and any physician can be asked to review the information in this book with you if you want to be sure your concerns are understood.

Understanding Nutrition Tables

SHARON'S STORY: *Learning About Nutrition*

Good nutrition and a healthy child certainly are a result of far more than X amount of iron or Y amount of protein, but the fact that nutrients can be quantified more easily than intangibles such as respect, love, and a stable home life means that nutrient data often form the main approach to scientific studies of health.

I must have seen the acronym "RDA" a million times on cereal boxes if nowhere else, but I had no idea how these Recommended Dietary Allowances were arrived at, or how a baby's requirements might differ from an adult's. I found the most recent (1974) booklet published by the National Academy of Sciences, which explains how the RDA's were developed and describes the research that determined these allowances. I was surprised to find out that even this prestigious group does not believe there are any absolutes in the field of nutrition; this lack of absolutes results in allowances for some nutrients being much higher or lower than might be right for any one individual.

• • •

Since 1941, the National Academy of Sciences has published nutritional guidelines known as the Recommended Dietary Allowances (RDA). Be careful not to confuse these with the United States Recommended Daily Allowances (U.S. RDA) which are based on the Recommended Dietary Allowances and used by the Food and Drug Administration for nutrition labeling.[9] More advanced guidelines called the Dietary Reference Intakes (DRI) are in the process of being formulated.

The most recently available nutritional recommendations for infants and children are given in the tables at the end of this chapter, as well as under individual entries in the nutrient sections below. Further updates to the new DRI are expected over the next few years. They can be obtained from your local library, your doctor or a nutritionist, or the National Academy Press in Washington, D.C.

Keep in mind that the numbers used by government officials and researchers for assessing the health of populations do not necessarily apply directly to individuals. If a given nutrient intake meets the needs of 98 percent of the population, many people obviously will need less than that amount. Therefore, while meeting the DRI for a particular nutrient is a good goal, falling a bit below that number won't necessarily result in malnutrition or poor health.

So what about babies? All babies obviously have the same basic nutritional requirements, whether or not they are vegetarians. The difference lies in how parents meet these requirements, always keeping in mind the individual needs of each child. You probably will be concerned about the amount of various foods your baby eats.

The National Academy recommends that beyond providing the individual nutrients, two additional guidelines should be followed: ". . . to ensure that possibly unrecognized nutritional needs are met, RDA should be provided from as varied a selection of foods as is practicable . . . [and] . . . as food has no nutritional value unless it is eaten, RDA should be provided from a selection of foods that are acceptable and palatable."[11]

As discussed above, with the exception of energy (calorie) requirements, DRIs are estimated to be larger than the average requirement in order to meet most people's nutritional needs over time. So if your child gets a bit less than the DRI, do not automatically assume your child is being malnourished, unless the child also seems chronically listless or sick. Also, a child's nutritional needs do vary from day to day, so minor omissions probably will be rectified within a short time. Learning and applying the general rules of good nutrition is far more important than trying to measure every bite your baby eats.

For children under one year of age, the DRI is based on the mean intake for healthy, breast-fed infants. The absorption of nutrients is sometimes less efficient in formulas than in breast milk; infant formulas, therefore, are required to contain higher amounts for many nutrients. For example: "A breast-fed infant receives about 60 milligrams of calcium per kilogram (300 milligrams/liter of milk) and retains about two-thirds of this. In contrast, an infant fed a standard cows' milk formula containing added calcium (600–700 milligrams of calcium per liter) receives about 170 milligrams of calcium per kilogram, but retains 25 to 30 percent. Although the breast-fed infant has less calcium available, its calcium needs are fully met by breast-feeding"[12]

The exception to basing nutritional requirements on breast milk occurs when research has shown that children become less healthy when supplemental foods are not added during the first year. Like cows' milk, human milk contains insufficient iron for a growing baby's needs after four to six months. Breast milk also contains insignificant amounts of vitamin D. These nutrients, therefore, must be provided in other ways. Supplemental vitamins and minerals, either in children's formulations or in fortified foods, are one possible answer, but whole grain cereals, green vegetables, dried fruits, molasses (for iron), and exposure to sunlight (for vitamin D) are valid alternatives in many cases. Let your child's response be your guide.

Remember that as solids are introduced into the diet, a mother's breast milk supply will decrease, and so the DRI must be met by a combination of solid food and breast milk. Also, if the mother's diet or health is poor, the breast milk supply may be deficient, in which case the baby will probably be hungry and "ask" for supplemental foods.

Meeting the Vegetarian Baby's Nutritional Needs

The key to raising a healthy vegetarian child is to have a good working knowledge of nutrition in general and vegetarian nutrition in particular, and to pay attention to areas where potential problems could arise. The following pages of this chapter contain detailed information about all the known nutrients, from vitamin A to zinc—information that will help you provide your baby with a well-rounded diet.

Macronutrients

ENERGY

RDA for energy (kilocalories/day)		
0 to 6 months: 650	6 to 12 months: 850	1 to 3 years: 1300

The energy your child needs to grow and explore is supplied by a combination of three types of nutrients: carbohydrates, proteins, and fats. Both carbohydrates and proteins supply four kilocalories per gram while fats contain nine kilocalories per gram.

The proportion of calories from carbohydrate, protein, and fat in a healthy baby's diet is substantially different from that recommended for older children and adults. On average, breast milk is 40 percent carbohydrate, 5 percent protein, 55 percent fat, and no fiber; while adults are told to eat (depending on the source) 50 to 80 percent carbohydrate, 10 to 20 percent protein, 10 to 30 percent fat, and a large amount of fiber. This means that throughout the first two years of life, and probably for some time beyond, your child will need considerably more fat and less fiber than you do.

When vegetarian children fail to thrive, the problem very often is one of not enough calories due to insufficient breast milk supply, premature weaning, inappropriate food selection, or inadequate meal frequency. By offering your child an abundance of energy-rich foods several times a day, difficulties stemming from too few calories can largely be prevented. (It should be noted, however, that breast-fed infants, in general, tend to grow somewhat more slowly than infants fed formula, and this difference in growth rate, so long as it remains normal, should not be mistaken for failure to thrive.) The white bread and fatty spread that might be a no-no for an adult can be just the thing to help a child grow.

On the other hand, you do not want to be so concerned about feeding your child enough food that you end up feeding too much. Obesity is a major problem in our society and has been linked to numerous diseases. Eating disorders are prevalent, as well. Respect your child's variable appetite level, and learn to both practice and teach the principles of self-demand feeding (discussed in chapter six) while also encouraging exercise and physical activity.

CARBOHYDRATES

RDA for carbohydrates: none established

Major vegetarian food sources for carbohydrates: grains, legumes, fruits, starchy vegetables, dairy products

Carbohydrates are the main energy source for human beings. Because infants and children need two to three times as much energy, per unit of body weight, as adults, carbohydrate-rich foods should form a substantial part of their diet.

Infants obtain plentiful carbohydrate from breast milk or formula. The main carbohydrate in breast milk is lactose, otherwise known as "milk sugar." According to La Leche League literature, "mothers' milk contains one-and-a-half times as much lactose as is found in cows' milk. . . ."[13] Formulas approximate breast milk by including either lactose (naturally present in cows' milk formulas) or other simple sugars such as sucrose.

Upon weaning, plant foods become the main source of carbohydrates in the diet although the lactose in dairy milk will continue to supply some energy for the child who eats dairy products. The main plant sources of carbohydrate energy in the toddler's diet are grains, legumes, fruits, and starchy vegetables. Other vegetables, nuts, and seeds also provide some carbohydrates.

Simple and Complex Carbohydrates

Carbohydrates are found in two basic types, simple and complex. Simple carbohydrates are the sugars and the sugar alcohols. The complex carbohydrates are starches, which are the storage form of glucose in plants; glycogen, the storage form of glucose in animals; and most types of fiber.[14]

Simple Carbohydrates

Sugars: glucose, fructose, galactose, lactose, sucrose, maltose, mannose, xylose

Sugar alcohols: sorbitol, mannitol, xylitol

Complex Carbohydrates

Starches: amylose, amylopectin

Fibers: cellulose, hemicellulose (including pectin and psyllium), lignin, mucilages, gums

Sugars and starches supply the calories your child needs while fibers promote proper digestive function and moderate blood sugar fluctuations. Too much fiber in a young child's diet can create problems, however, so a high fiber diet is inappropriate for the first years of life. Since the body needs B-complex vitamins for proper energy metabolism, make sure to use fortified products when feeding your child refined grain products such as white rice, white pasta, white bread, and cold cereals. Such foods will probably make up a relatively small portion of your child's diet, however, and with whole foods, especially whole grains, the need for fortification of B-complex vitamins is reduced or eliminated.

PROTEINS

RDA for protein (grams/day)

0 to 6 months: 13	6 to 12 months: 14	1 to 3 years: 16

Major vegetarian food sources for protein: whole grains, legumes, vegetables, nuts, seeds, seitan, soy products, dairy products, eggs

As long as children's energy needs are being met they will thrive on a diet in which protein is available from a mixture of plant foods.

Gil Langley[16]

Protein is the essential building block of all body tissues, including cell walls, muscles, blood, hair, and internal organs such as the heart and brain, as well as being used in the formation of hormones, enzymes, and antibodies. Protein also can serve as a source of energy if carbohydrate and fat intake are for some reason not high enough to meet these needs. Use of protein as a major energy source may stress the kidneys, however, so protein should not be oversupplied in the diet at the expense of the other macronutrients.

Since babies are growing so rapidly, they need more protein per unit of body weight than do adults, who need it primarily for maintaining their fully developed tissues. Babies under six months need three times as much protein per pound of body weight as do adults; between six months and a year, children need twice as much; after one year, that drops to one-and-one-half times the adult requirement. To give you some idea of the rate at which a baby grows, note that according to the National Academy of Sciences a baby adds "about 3.5 grams [of body protein] a day during the first four months and 3.1 grams per day during the next eight months."[17] A consistent supply of dietary protein is, therefore, essential to your child's steady growth.

Protein is composed of amino acids. There are 22 amino acids that must be brought together in order to make human proteins. Fourteen of these amino acids are produced by the body, but the remaining eight, called essential amino acids, must be supplied by the diet. For babies and children, one, and possibly two, other semi-essential amino acids must be included in the diet during growth periods.[18] Note that non-dairy infant formula should be supplemented with the non-essential amino acid carnitine as infants may be unable to synthesize enough of this protein when they are rapidly growing.[19] Taurine also is added to soy formula.[20]

Amino Acids

Essential Amino Acids: isoleucine, leucine, lysine, threonine, tryptophan, valine, methionine, phenylalanine

Semi-essential Amino Acids (essential only for growing children): arginine, histidine

The RDA for protein for the first six months of life was determined from an analysis of the milk of lactating mothers. Thus, so long as a baby is primarily breast-fed, or given a quality formula, there will be no problem obtaining sufficient amounts of protein with the proper amounts and ratios of the essential amino acids. From six months of age on, the RDA is based on an analysis of omnivorous milk-and-solid diets of thriving babies. The RDA for protein should, therefore, be adequate for lacto-ovo vegetarian children, but it may not be correct for vegan babies which is why it might be wise to continue breast-feeding vegan children well into their second year.

In the past, it was thought that animal foods supplied all the essential amino acids in approximately the right proportions for human health while plant foods were "incomplete," meaning they were grossly deficient in, or even completely lacking, one or more of the essential amino acids. As a result, vegetarian adults not only laboriously "combined proteins" at every meal, but were told that their vegetarian, and especially vegan, children were at grave risk of protein deficiency.

More study and debate has resulted in a different conclusion. It now is recognized that plants do indeed contain all the essential amino acids and so the labels "complete" and "incomplete" are misleading. Instead, foods now are rated according to protein "digestibility" using data for 2- to 5-year-old children.[21] Digestibility is determined not only by the amino acid profile of the food, but also includes factors for food constituents that affect protein absorption such as fiber, tannins, and phytates.[22] (Note that several chemicals naturally present in foods are suspected of hindering the absorption of certain nutrients. Tannins are phenolic compounds commonly found in coffee and black tea which greatly reduce non-heme iron absorption. Phytates are salts formed from the phytic acid in plants, especially cereal grains, and they bind with minerals such as calcium, iron, magnesium, copper, and zinc. Another calcium-binding substance is oxalate, a salt of oxalic acid, which is found in "high-oxalate" vegetables such as Swiss chard, spinach, beet greens, and rhubarb.)[23-24]

The term "quality" still is used in reference to protein digestibility, and except for isolated soy protein, plant foods tend to have lower ratings than animal foods. Even so, plants easily can meet protein needs even for young children if they are eaten in sufficient quantity and variety. Parents should, however, keep in mind that although vegetarian adults and older children need not consciously combine protein-rich foods, the theory of protein combining still may have some value for very young children during and after weaning, especially for children weaned well before the age of two years.[25] This is due to a combination of factors such as the rapidity of a young child's growth, and subsequent higher need for certain amino acids, coupled with a less robust digestive system and a small stomach that is not capable of accepting large quantities of food at any one time.

To give an example of protein combining, legumes are, in general, relatively low in (but not "lacking!" *see Table 2.3, page 101*) methionine, while grains are lower in threonine and lysine.[26] Combining legumes and grains at a meal thus results in a good mixture of amino acids all entering the digestive tract at the same time. Some protein-enhancing food combinations are listed below.

1. grains with legumes
2. grains with nuts or seeds
3. legumes with nuts or seeds
4. dairy products (including breast milk or formula) with grains, legumes, nuts, or seeds
5. eggs with grains, legumes, nuts, or seeds

Obviously, these combinations occur naturally in the preparation of common foods such as rice and bean burritos, lentil-nut loafs, nut-butter sandwiches, macaroni and cheese, and scrambled eggs on toast. Add in some breast milk or, in the diet of the older child, soy drink, and your child easily will receive a full range of essential amino acids. Total protein intake will not be a problem so long as total calorie needs are being met.

RDA for fat: none established

Major vegetarian food sources for fat: avocados, olives, nuts, seeds, oils, whole-fat soy products, whole-fat dairy products, egg yolks

Major vegetarian food sources for alpha-linolenic (omega-3) essential fatty acid: ground flax seeds, pumpkin seeds, walnuts, whole-fat soy products, flaxseed oil, canola oil, walnut oil, soybean oil, hempseed oil

Fats are the most concentrated form of energy for the body, supplying over twice the calories per gram of carbohydrates or proteins. This high concentration of calories make fats a valuable source of energy for babies which is undoubtedly why breast milk contains such a large percentage of calories as fat. Breast milk or formula will provide the fat an infant needs and will continue to be an important source of fat until the child is weaned.

As your child grows, the percentage of fat in his or her diet should gradually be decreased as excessive amounts of fat can contribute to the development of obesity, but very low fat diets definitely are contraindicated for children during the first two years of life and probably well beyond. Fat not only supplies the energy a growing child needs but is important for absorption of the fat-soluble vitamins, A, D, E, and K.

Keep in mind that not all fats are created equal. Saturated fats and trans-fatty acids have been linked to cardiovascular disease while excessive amounts of polyunsaturated fats have been linked to cancer.[27-28] And the "fake" fats, such as Olean, being added to convenience foods can drain nutrients from the body while creating such distressing intestinal disturbances as abdominal cramps.

In addition, a small percentage of the fats in whole foods are in the form of the two essential fatty acids (EFA): linoleic acid (omega-6) and alpha-linolenic acid (omega-3), the latter of which is especially important for proper formation and continued health of the brain and central nervous system. The ideal proportion is thought to be around 3 percent of calories from omega-6 fatty acids and 1 percent from omega-3 fatty acids, a ratio of 3:1, but omnivorous Americans eat a diet with a ratio closer to 20:1, and vegetarian diets can be even more unbalanced.

The best way to include fats in your child's diet is to offer whole or lightly processed foods that contain a reasonable portion of mostly unsaturated fats, including some rich in omega-3 fatty acids. When cooking and making salad dressings, choose olive, canola, and flax oils over safflower, sunflower, and corn oils. Your child's growth pattern, as well as energy and hunger levels, are your best guides in determining the amount of fatty foods to offer.

Micronutrients

Vitamins and minerals do not provide energy but are needed to form the enzymes that allow energy production and other metabolic processes to occur. The following nutrients certainly are essential to growth and proper functioning, and most of them are amply supplied by most diets, including vegetarian ones. Vegetarian children who eat whole foods, rather than empty calorie "junk" foods, might even be less likely to exhibit deficiencies of some these nutrients than are children who consume many processed foods.

The micronutrients to pay the most attention to in the diet of your vegetarian baby are vitamin D, vitamin B-12, calcium, iron, and zinc.

Fat-Soluble Vitamins

VITAMIN A

RDA for vitamin A (micrograms RE/day):
 0 to 6 months: 375   6 to 12 months: 375   1 to 3 years: 400

Major vegetarian food sources of vitamin A: vegetables, fruits, dairy products, eggs

Vitamin A helps fight infection and inflammation; helps build skin, bones, teeth, hair, and other tissues; and is needed for good eyesight and night vision. It also is used in the synthesis of RNA, the genetic material which in turn synthesizes cellular protein, and assists in hormonal and reproductive functioning. Because young children have not yet developed large stores of vitamin A in their own tissues, foods rich in vitamin A should be offered regularly.

Two kinds of vitamin A are found in natural sources. Pre-formed vitamin A (retinol and related compounds) is found in animal fats. Because it is stored in fat tissues, pre-formed vitamin A can be toxic if ingested in very large amounts. The other type is pro-vitamin A, a subset of the approximately 600 carotenes found in plants. Beta-carotene is the most active of these precursors which are converted to vitamin A in the body, with alpha- and gamma-carotenes also exhibiting good activity. The carotenes are non-toxic, even in large amounts, and may protect against cancer. Vitamin A usually is listed in terms of Retinol Equivalents (RE) to take into account the difference between pre-formed and pro-vitamin A.

Over cooking and long storage of vegetables decrease the availability of vitamin A, but light steaming can increase the bioavailability of carotenoids as can the addition of some fat to the dish.[29] Vitamin A function also requires the presence of other vitamins (B-complex, C, D, and E) and minerals (calcium, phosphorus, and zinc).

VITAMIN D

DRI for vitamin D (micrograms/day)		
0 to 6 months: 5	6 to 12 months: 5	1 to 3 years: 5

Major vegetarian food sources of vitamin D: fortified foods

Modern humans . . . have less sun exposure as a result of urbanization, smog, greater population density at northern latitudes, and less time spent outdoors.

Mark and Virginia Messina[30]

Vitamin D is essential for the absorption of calcium, which is one reason it commonly is added to cows' milk, and to some soy milks, as well. The body also needs vitamin D to assimilate phosphorus, which is used in teeth and bone formation. A reliable vitamin D source, therefore, is essential to proper development of the skeleton in growing children.

For vegetarians, vitamin D comes from a vitamin supplement or fortified foods, or it is formed in the body upon exposure of the skin (without sunscreen) to the ultraviolet rays of the sun. A little vitamin D can go a long way, and adults seem to be able to store enough vitamin D during sunny, warm weather to supply their own needs through the winter. But given the damage that can be caused by a vitamin D deficiency, don't depend solely on body stores to get your child through the winter months.[31]

Only a trace of vitamin D is naturally present in breast milk, but it is not clear that this is a problem for breast-fed infants.[32] However, if your baby is born in the winter months, you rarely go outside, you live in an area that tends towards cloudiness even in warm weather, or your baby has dark skin, you should ask your doctor about supplementation for your infant while nursing.

Keep in mind that an overdose of supplemental vitamin D can be toxic, so as you wean your child be careful not to exceed the DRI from supplements and fortified foods.[33] Also, the DRI assumes "the absence of adequate exposure to sunlight," so you are probably safe to give your child little or no supplementation during sunny weather if your baby goes outside much. This does not mean exposing your child to a potentially dangerous amount of sunlight, but instead entails going out in the morning or late afternoon for 15 minutes (light skin) to 30 minutes (dark skin) of direct, warm sunlight on the face and hands every day, a task easily accomplished by a half-hour of play in the park or a short walk.

VITAMIN E

RDA for vitamin E (milligrams α-TE/day)

0 to 6 months: 3	6 to 12 months: 4	1 to 3 years: 6

Major vegetarian food sources for vitamin E: whole grains, nuts, seeds, olive oil, sunflower oil, sweet potatoes, cabbage, green leafy vegetables

The most important function of vitamin E is protecting the body from the damaging effects of oxidation, especially within cellular membranes. Oxidation is a process by which chemicals called "free radicals" bind with cell membranes and proteins, thereby damaging them. By reducing the number of free radicals circulating in the body, the anti-oxidant vitamin E aids the healing process and helps protect against a host of degenerative conditions later in life. With ample vitamin E intake, wounds heal more completely, the muscles of the body function more efficiently, and the aging process may even be slowed.

Vegetarian diets are high in vitamin E but also can be high in the polyunsaturated fatty acids which oxidize and then must be removed from the body through the action of vitamin E. The very best sources of this nutrient, therefore, are whole foods which are high in vitamin E but low in polyunsaturated fats.

Although vitamin E is fat soluble, the body excretes it quickly so overdoses are rare.

VITAMIN K

RDA for vitamin K (micrograms/day)

0 to 6 months: 5	6 to 12 months: 10	1 to 3 years: 15

Major vegetarian food sources for vitamin K: green leafy vegetables, legumes, soybean oil, canola oil, olive oil

Vitamin K is vital for proper blood clotting through the production of prothrombin and other proteins that regulate blood coagulation. Vitamin K also helps form proteins in the bones and kidneys.

Vitamin K is found in two forms, one produced by plants (vitamin K-1) and the other by bacteria (vitamin K-2), including organisms found in the human colon. Because vitamin K is amply available in foods, deficiencies are rare in adults, but newborn infants often need a supplement and so generally are given an injection of vitamin K at the time of birth. In addition, a vitamin K supplement might be needed for a breast-fed infant or a baby who has suffered a blood loss or who must take oral antibiotics.

Water-soluble Vitamins

VITAMIN B-COMPLEX

DRI for Vitamin B-1 (Thiamin) (milligrams/day)
0 to 6 months: 0.2   6 to 12 months: 0.3   1 to 3 years: 0.5

DRI for Vitamin B-2 (Riboflavin) (milligrams/day)
0 to 6 months: 0.3   6 to 12 months: 0.4   1 to 3 years: 0.5

DRI for Vitamin B-3 (Niacin) (milligrams NE/day)
0 to 6 months: 2   6 to 12 months: 4   1 to 3 years: 6

DRI for Vitamin B-6 (Pyridoxine) (milligrams/day)
0 to 6 months: 0.1   6 to 12 months: 0.3   1 to 3 years: 0.5

DRI for Biotin (micrograms/day)
0 to 6 months: 5   6 to 12 months: 6   1 to 3 years: 8

DRI for Choline (milligrams/day)
0 to 6 months: 125   6 to 12 months: 150   1 to 3 years: 200

DRI for Folate (micrograms DFE/day)
0 to 6 months: 65   6 to 12 months: 80   1 to 3 years: 150

DRI for Pantothenic Acid (milligrams/day)
0 to 6 months: 1.7   6 to 12 months: 1.8   1 to 3 years: 2

Major vegetarian food sources of vitamin B-complex: sea
vegetables, dairy products, eggs, whole grains, legumes, tempeh,
nuts, seeds, green leafy vegetables, mushrooms, avocados,
fortified foods (*Note:* The individual foods in this list do not
necessarily each contain high amounts of all B vitamins, but a
diet that contains a variety of foods from this list should
contain a full range of the B-complex.)

The B vitamins are grouped together as "B-complex" because
each seems to be essential to the proper functioning of the
others. In whole foods, they tend all to be present together in
varying proportions, so if a person is eating a variety of whole
foods, deficiencies of B vitamins are unlikely. The only major
exception is vitamin B-12 which is discussed in detail below.

The B vitamins are essential to the proper functioning of the nervous, cardiovascular, and enzymatic systems. They also are necessary for the metabolism of carbohydrates, fats, and proteins. Because they are delicate and water-soluble, soaking in water and cooking can destroy many of the B-complex vitamins. The body also eliminates them rapidly, so foods rich in B vitamins should be offered to your child daily.

Sea vegetables, whole grains, and fortified nutritional yeast are excellent sources of the B-complex vitamins. The paucity of whole foods in the standard American diet is one reason it tends to be low in B vitamins. A vegetarian diet, on the other hand, often includes many raw and lightly cooked whole plant foods and so is more likely to be adequate.

Special note: Goats' milk is very low in folacin, so if you feed your child goats' milk, either use a fortified product or be sure to include foods rich in folic acid in the diet. In the past, powdered goats' milk formulas also were reported as being deficient in pyridoxine (vitamin B-6), so be sure to use a fortified product if that is what you feed your infant.[34]

VITAMIN B-12

DRI for Vitamin B-12 (Cyanocobalamin) (micrograms/day)
  0 to 6 months: 0.4   6 to 12 months: 0.5   1 to 3 years: 0.9

Major vegetarian food sources for vitamin B-12: dairy products, egg yolks, fortified foods

Vitamin B-12 is the general name for a group of substances called cobalamins which are vital for cell division, especially of the red blood cells, as well as the maintenance of a healthy nervous system. Unfortunately for vegans and near-vegans, this is the one nutrient that is impossible to obtain reliably from plant foods in the modern world.

The reason is that vitamin B-12 is synthesized by bacteria and other microorganisms. In nature, herbivorous animals eat plants and drink water which are contaminated by insects and microorganisms and which, as a result, supply this vitamin. Some animals also absorb vitamin B-12 manufactured by the microorganisms naturally present in their intestines. Furthermore, they then pass those B-12-producing organisms through their feces back into the environment, a process that has even been theorized to apply to humans living in primitive conditions.[35]

The modern sanitation practices which have resulted in so many health benefits also have reduced microbial contamination to such low levels that vegetarians who eat little or no dairy products and eggs cannot depend on such sources for this vitamin even if they eat organically grown plant foods. This is especially true for babies as they don't have large body stores of this vitamin as do many adults who become vegan later in life. The solution is not to add contaminated food and water to your family's diet, but instead to regularly include supplements or foods which are fortified with vitamin B-12.

Some vegetarians resist all supplementation, but in this case it is vital for your health and your baby's. Folic acid, which is very available in plant foods, can mask a B-12 deficiency so that irreversible nerve damage can occur long before the development of pernicious anemia makes a B-12 deficiency obvious. Furthermore, vitamin B-12 analogs (found in foods such as sea vegetables, spirulina, miso, and tempeh, and confused in the past with true vitamin B-12, due to inaccurate laboratory tests) appear to interfere with the action of cobalamin in the body.[36] Reliance on seaweeds as a source of B-12 is not recommended.[37]

Fortunately, vitamin B-12 is only needed—even by children—in very small amounts, easily supplied by common vegetarian products such as fortified soy milk, fortified cereals, and fortified nutritional yeast. Pregnant and nursing women should include a reliable B-12 source in their diet (see page 106), while children should be given a supplement or fortified foods after they are no longer nursing substantially. A tablespoon of Red Star Vegetarian Support Formula (T6635) nutritional yeast supplies the DRI for all B vitamins, including vitamin B-12. But don't assume other yeasts contain B-12, and be aware that labels on some products such as spirulina may be out of date with regard to vitamin

B-12. If you are unsure, contact the manufacturer to make sure they are adding cyanocobalamin to their product.

VITAMIN C (ASCORBIC ACID)

RDA for vitamin C (milligrams/day)

0 to 6 months: 30	6 to 12 months: 35	1 to 3 years: 40

Major vegetarian food sources for vitamin C: citrus fruits, berries, melons, guava, papaya, kiwi, pineapple, tomatoes, potatoes, bell peppers, leafy green vegetables

Vitamin C is an anti-oxidant which protects the body from free radical damage. In addition, vitamin C is necessary for the formation and maintenance of connective tissue (collagen), and aids the metabolism of proteins and the synthesis of hormones, helps eliminate excess cholesterol from the body, and facilitates the utilization of other nutrients, including iron. For growing children, vitamin C is necessary for the formation of strong teeth and gums.

Almost any fresh, raw fruit will provide ample amounts of vitamin C. Vegetables, both raw and lightly cooked, also provide large amounts. Because vitamin C is used quickly and can't be stored by the body, it should be a part of most meals.

Cooking, cutting, or bruising produce consumes vitamin C fairly quickly because this vitamin is destroyed by contact with oxygen. To minimize this loss, handle produce carefully, cook vegetables quickly, and feed your child fresh, raw produce, especially fruits, or freshly made juices.

Vitamin C is rarely a toxic in adults, but large doses of supplemental vitamin C can cause problems for children, including erosion of tooth enamel if the supplement is in the form of chewable tablets. Since fresh fruit is usually a favorite with babies, vitamin C is easily supplied in a vegetarian diet, and there should be no need for supplementation.

Major Minerals

The following minerals are called "major" or "macro" minerals, not because of their action in the body, but because they compose at least 0.01 percent of the body's weight and must be included in the diet in relatively large quantities.[38]

CALCIUM

DRI for Calcium (milligrams/day)

  0 to 6 months: 210   6 to 12 months: 270   1 to 3 years: 500

Major vegetarian food sources for calcium: dairy products, low-oxalate green leafy vegetables (kale, broccoli, Brussels sprouts, turnip greens, cabbage), sea vegetables, soy products (including calcium-precipitated tofu), legumes, nuts, seeds, dried fruits (especially figs), blackstrap molasses, fortified foods

Lacto-ovo vegetarians have calcium intakes that are comparable to or higher than those of non-vegetarians . . . [and] vegans may have lower calcium needs than non-vegetarians because diets that are low in total protein and more alkaline have been shown to have a calcium-sparing effect.

Virginia Messina and Kenneth Burke[39]

Calcium is the most plentiful mineral in the human body and is found primarily in bones and teeth with small amounts (less than one percent) in blood and soft tissues. In combination with magnesium, calcium helps maintain a healthy heart, and it also aids in muscle growth and assists in muscle contraction and relaxation. Calcium is essential in the diets of young babies, even before birth, not only for growth of the muscular-skeleton system, but also since some teeth begin forming around the fourth or fifth month of pregnancy. A deficiency of calcium during this time cannot be reversed, but once formed, the calcium in teeth tends to be stable.[40]

Calcium balance, which is the net effect of absorption and excretion, generally is a better indicator of calcium status than is calcium intake alone. Vitamin D, magnesium, phosphorus, and perhaps boron, are needed for proper absorption and utilization of calcium by the body. Weight-bearing exercise is another vital factor for the formation and maintenance of strong bones. On the other hand, excessive protein, iron, phosphorus (generally from soft drinks), and sodium can contribute to loss of calcium from the body, as can caffeine (which in a child's diet means soft drinks, tea, and chocolate), tobacco smoke (for children, secondhand smoke), and a sedentary lifestyle.

Total absorption rates for dietary calcium range from 30 to 40 percent, a factor which is used when making recommendations.[41] Relatively low dietary intake of calcium can result in increased absorption by the body, and infants can absorb as much as three-quarters of the calcium they eat, but don't rely on this mechanism for your child. Instead, strive to include plenty of calcium-rich foods in your child's diet.[42]

Breast milk (or formula) supplies all the calcium a baby needs in the first six months of life and continues to supply a substantial amount through the months of weaning. After weaning, lacto-vegetarian children will continue to obtain much of their calcium from dairy products, but by making combinations of foods, such as vegetable-legume soups and tofu-smoothies, you can supply your child's need for this nutrient from calcium-rich plants alone. You would be wise to include some calcium-fortified foods, however, especially if your child has a small appetite or is a picky eater. Fortified orange juice or soy milk are excellent choices that are likely to be well received.

CHLORIDE

ESADDI for Chloride (milligrams/day)
0 to 6 months: 180   6 to 12 months: 300   1 to 2 years: 350
2 to 3 years: 500

Major vegetarian food sources for chloride: salt, plants, dairy products

Chloride is distributed throughout the body, mostly in fluids such as blood. It helps regulate the acid-alkaline balance of the body and is used in various metabolic processes such as transport of carbon dioxide and maintenance of connective tissue. Because chloride is so readily available in foods, it need not be consciously added to your child's diet. The only exception is infant formula which now is required to be fortified with this mineral due to problems with deficiency in the past.

The chloride found in foods such as salt (sodium chloride) is bound with other substances and is the form the body metabolizes. The free chlorine found in chlorinated water and household bleach should not be confused with dietary chloride.

MAGNESIUM

DRI for Magnesium (milligrams/day)

0 to 6 months: 30   6 to 12 months: 75   1 to 3 years: 80

Major vegetarian food sources for magnesium: whole grains, legumes, nuts, dark green vegetables, dairy products, eggs

Magnesium is needed for many metabolic processes such as energy production, protein synthesis, excretion of excess ammonia, formation of tooth enamel, and proper functioning of the nervous, musculo-skeletal, and immune systems. Magnesium also is a vital component for potassium retention in the cells.

Like calcium, approximately 30 to 40 percent of dietary magnesium is absorbed. The rate of magnesium absorption is reduced by fat, calcium, phosphorus, lactose, phytate, and oxalate, and enhanced by eating magnesium-rich foods over the course of the day rather than only at one meal or through a supplement.

PHOSPHORUS

DRI for Phosphorus (milligrams/day)

0 to 6 months: 100   6 to 12 months: 275   1 to 3 years: 460

Major vegetarian food sources for phosphorus: dairy products, eggs, whole grains, legumes, fruits

Phosphorus is found in every cell of the body with the majority being bound with calcium in the skeleton in the form of calcium phosphate. Phosphorus is fundamental to the formation of nucleic acids and proteins, energy metabolism, and the activation of the B-complex vitamins. As with calcium, vitamin D is needed for the absorption of phosphorus.

The phosphorus-calcium ratio is important to bone health. Formerly, it was recommended that this ratio be around one-to-one

(1:1) in adults, and no greater than two-to-one (2:1), especially for diets low in calcium. The new DRIs recommend slightly more calcium than phosphorus. Soft drinks and many other junk foods contain large amounts of phosphorus, and little or no calcium, which can drastically skew the balance of those two nutrients. Your child will benefit from avoiding such foods.

POTASSIUM

EMR for Potassium (milligrams/day)

0 to 6 months: 500   6 to 12 months: 700   1 to 2 year: 1000

2 to 3 years: 1400

Major vegetarian food sources for potassium: fruits, grains, vegetables

Potassium is a key mineral, vital in combination with sodium. The vast majority of potassium is found inside the cells with small amounts in extra-cellular fluids. Energy metabolism, blood pressure regulation, and the transmission of impulses along the nerves all depend upon this mineral.

Potassium is very easily absorbed by the body and is unlikely to be deficient unless an individual is starved, dehydrated, or severely stressed by surgery or illness. An adequate body store of magnesium is also essential for maintaining proper potassium levels by preventing potassium excretion.

SODIUM

EMR for Sodium (milligrams/day)

0 to 6 months: 120   6 to 12 months: 200   1 to 2 years: 225

2 to 3 years: 300

Major vegetarian food sources for sodium: salt, dairy products, eggs, soy sauce, pickled vegetables, baking soda, baking powder, sodium-based food additives, softened water

Although most adolescents and adults would benefit from less salt in their diet, it would be inappropriate to restrict salt sharply in the infant and growing child.

The Yale Guide to Children's Nutrition[43]

Sodium is found predominantly in the spaces between the cells where it works with potassium to regulate the fluid concentrations and the sources of energy metabolism, blood pressure stability, and the transmission of nerve impulses.

While infants and toddlers should not have their salt intake restricted, neither is there any reason to include excessive amounts of sodium in your child's diet. Most young children prefer bland foods and so will be unlikely to eat too much sodium unless they are fed a diet high in processed foods. Since a taste for salty foods can develop from childhood eating patterns, a moderation of salt intake is appropriate when your child begins school.

Trace Minerals

The trace, or "micro," minerals are those which compose less than 0.01 percent of the body's weight. Most of these are readily available in the diet and so will not be discussed in detail. You might note that, in large amounts, many trace minerals tend to be toxic which is why mineral supplements beyond a standard daily vitamin/mineral should generally only be used when necessary to treat a diagnosed condition or deficiency.

If your family obtains a large amount of food from home-grown and local crops, make sure the local soil has a good supply of minerals so the plants contain everything you need. (Also check for undesirable elements like lead.) Iodine, selenium, and zinc are examples of minerals that can be lacking in some areas, so if your family's diet is limited to local foods, deficiencies are more likely to develop. By including foods that were grown in other areas, or taking care to add minerals to the soil of your garden, this is less likely. Contact your local agricultural service for information on local soils, testing procedures, and amendments.

Water also can contribute trace minerals to the diet depending on the source and processing procedures.

Trace Minerals

Arsenic, boron, chromium, cobalt, copper, fluoride, iodine, iron, manganese, molybdenum, nickel, selenium, silicon, tin, vanadium, zinc

COPPER

Major vegetarian food sources for copper: whole grains, legumes, nuts, seeds, green leafy vegetables, mushrooms, eggs

Copper is important in a variety of enzymatic functions and contributes to the health of the skeletal, nervous, and cardiovascular systems. Copper helps absorb and mobilize iron, and copper deficiency can accompany iron-deficiency anemia. Copper also assists the conversion of alpha-linolenic (omega 3) fatty acid into longer chain fatty acids such as EPA and DHA.[44]

The absorption of copper is reduced by vitamin C, calcium, phosphorus, and niacin, and possibly by large amounts of fiber and phytates. Because these nutrients are well supplied by vegetarian diets, some concern has been expressed about copper absorption in vegetarians. Vegetarian diets tend to contain larger amounts of copper than standard American diets, however, and lower amounts of its antagonist, zinc, so lower absorption rates appear to be fairly well balanced by the increased intake.

You will want to make sure your child eats a diet which contains copper-rich foods that are lower in those substances which hinder absorption. Nuts, seeds, mushrooms, and eggs are especially good choices. Absorption might be enhanced if these foods sometimes are eaten as isolated snacks, separate from other foods high in vitamin C, calcium, and so on. Copper pots and copper plumbing also can increase dietary copper levels.

FLUORIDE

Major vegetarian food sources for fluoride: fluoridated water (either natural or supplemented), foods prepared with such water, foods prepared in Teflon-coated pans, tea

Fluoride has been recognized as the single most influential factor responsible for the observed decline in caries in children as well as adults.[45]

Fluoride (an anion of the element fluorine) is not considered to be an essential nutrient, but it might contribute to bone health, and it definitely helps children develop strong teeth that are resistant to decay. Not only can fluoride be incorporated into tooth enamel during the formative years (up to age seven), but the continued presence of fluoride in the diet decreases the rate of tooth demineralization and increases the rate of remineralization, thus preserving the enamel and preventing the development of dental caries.

Concern has been raised by some members of the alternative health community regarding the potential toxicity of fluoride. As with many nutrients, and especially minerals, excessive amounts of fluoride can create problems, the most obvious being a discoloration of the teeth known as fluorosis. But rather than avoid this mineral altogether, you just need to make sure all the sources of fluoride in your child's diet are taken into account. Your child's pediatrician and dentist should know how much fluoride is in your local tap water and your child's toothpaste, for example, and any supplements they prescribe will then be based upon those numbers. For that reason, it is important that you let them know if you use filtered water, well water, or fluoride-free toothpaste.

IODINE

RDA for iodine (micrograms/day)

| 0 to 6 months: 40 | 6 to 12 months: 50 | 1 to 3 years: 70 |

Major vegetarian food sources for iodine: plants grown in iodine-rich soil, sea vegetables, iodized salt

Iodine is necessary for the proper functioning of the thyroid gland, which regulates growth, development, and metabolic rate. The healthy range for iodine intake is rather narrow, and either chronically deficient or excessive amounts of this mineral can create thyroid dysfunction and related health problems.

A diet which contains a wide variety of plant foods which were, in turn, grown on a wide variety of soils, and which also includes some sea vegetables and a judicious amount of iodized salt, should supply all the iodine your child needs.

IRON

RDA for iron (milligrams/day)

0 to 6 months: 6   6 to 12 months: 10   1 to 3 years: 10

Major vegetarian food sources for iron: sea vegetables, whole grains, legumes, nuts, seeds, dried fruits, green leafy vegetables, blackstrap molasses, egg yolks, foods cooked in cast-iron pans, fortified foods

Among the measures to be taken [to prevent iron deficiency anemia] are . . . the advocation of exclusive breast-feeding up to 6 months of age, discouraging the use of fresh cows' milk at least up to month 9 of life, the use of iron-fortified infant formulas when formulas are used, the inclusion of foods that facilitate iron absorption in the diet, . . . and iron supplementation.[46]

Iron is essential in the production of healthy blood. It works with protein and copper to produce hemoglobin, which carries oxygen from the lungs to the tissues, and myoglobin, which supplies oxygen to the muscle cells.

If the mother has a good iron supply and the baby is full term, there is usually no need to supplement a breast milk diet with iron until after four to six months. Delaying the clamping of the umbilical cord during the seconds immediately after birth can significantly increase the baby's initial iron stores, but the huge volume of fluid which is transferred to the baby by such a delay also can cause respiratory and circulatory problems. You, therefore, will want to discuss the timing of cord-clamping with your doctor or midwife.[47] If the child is premature, or the mother has a low iron reading during pregnancy, the stores of iron that a baby is born with will be much lower than otherwise. Premature babies probably will be given iron supplementation.

After four to six months, the baby's blood mass has increased to the point where iron must be added. At this point, iron-rich foods should be introduced to the diet. Low iron levels are not caused by a vegetarian diet, but "can affect children regardless of the kind of diet they eat—omnivore, lacto-ovo vegetarian, or vegan."[48]

Current nutritional theory recommends, for all ages, levels of iron intake that are difficult to meet without a supplement or fortified foods. It should be noted, however, that iron supplements are a fairly recent development. It is possible that previous generations' use of iron-rich wild greens and iron pots for cooking (rather than the aluminum and non-stick ones commonly used today), may have provided sufficient iron for good health The iron content of foods can be significantly increased by cooking with iron skillets and pots, so you may want to purchase a few for your kitchen.[49] Stainless steel cookware can increase the iron content of some foods as well.[50]

The ascorbic acid (vitamin C), malic acid, and citric acid found in fruits and vegetables enhance iron absorption by helping to change ferric iron into ferrous iron, which is more efficiently used by the body. As an example, the iron content in foods such as egg yolks and cereal grains is high, but it is in the form of ferric iron. The American tradition of drinking orange juice with breakfast, therefore, can improve the iron absorption from these common breakfast foods.

On the other hand, phytates and tannins can interfere with iron absorption, and according to the authors of *The Dietitian's Guide to Vegetarian Diets*, "the calcium in dairy products can markedly inhibit iron absorption. The addition of modest amounts of milk or cheese to a meal of pizza or hamburger has been shown to reduce the iron absorption by 50 to 60 percent."[51] Therefore, dairy products should be fed to your child separately from iron-rich foods.

MANGANESE

ESADDI for Manganese (milligrams/day)

0 to 6 months: 0.3 to 0.6	6 to 12 months: 0.6 to 1.0
1 to 3 years: 1.0 to 1.5	

Major vegetarian food sources for manganese: whole grains,
legumes, nuts, sweet potatoes, pineapple, spices, and tea

Manganese is important in carbohydrate and fat synthesis, bone
and skin formation, and prevention of damage from the oxidation
of fats. It is adversely affected by iron, phosphorus, phytates,
fiber, calcium, and copper.

MOLYBDENUM

ESADDI for Molybdenum (micrograms/day)
0 to 6 months: 15 to 30   6 to 12 month: 20 to 40
1 to 3 years: 25 to 50

Major vegetarian food sources for molybdenum: whole grains,
legumes, green leafy vegetables, dairy products

Molybdenum is used in the manufacture of enzymes. Many
foods contain large amounts of this mineral (for example, a quarter cup of lima beans contains 150 micrograms), so it is plenti-
fully supplied by a whole foods diet.

SELENIUM

RDA for selenium (micrograms/day)
0 to 6 months 10   6 to 12 months 15   1 to 3 years 20

Major vegetarian food sources for selenium: grains, legumes,
nuts (especially Brazils), seeds, mushrooms, eggs

Selenium is an essential nutrient. . . . It is present in many . . .
grains, and legumes, but amounts vary according to the soil content in which the food . . . was grown.[52]

Selenium is a factor in thyroid function and also helps form
enzymes which work to prevent oxidative damage. The amount
of selenium in a plant-based diet is directly related to the amount
present in the soil in which the plants were grown, varying by as
much as a thousand fold between growing regions.[53] As was mentioned above in the entry for iodine, it is important to eat plants
that were grown in a wide variety of soils. If your family eats
mostly local produce, test your soil and amend as indicated.

ZINC

RDA for zinc (milligrams/day)

0 to 6 months: 5   6 to 12 months: 5   1 to 3 years: 10

Major vegetarian food sources for zinc: whole grains, wheat germ, sea vegetables, green leafy vegetables, corn, green peas, potatoes, mushrooms, legumes, soy products, nuts, seeds, dairy products, egg yolks, fortified foods

Vegetarian zinc intake is similar or somewhat lower than non-vegetarian intake, and the absorption of zinc from plants is somewhat lower than from animal products. The zinc RDA is a subject of debate, however, and some researchers believe that it may be higher than necessary.[54]

Zinc is an important trace mineral that is often forgotten in the diet. Found in all the cells of the body, zinc is vital for proper enzymatic, nervous, and immune function. Zinc-rich foods must be eaten daily as body stores are not readily accessible.

Your child needs plenty of zinc to achieve normal growth as it is necessary for blood formation, protein synthesis, and cell replication. The American Academy of Pediatrics does not recommend zinc supplements, however, since ". . . clinical signs of [zinc] deficiency are rare among vegetarians."[55] This might be a result of the fact that the need for zinc increases with protein intake, so the lower protein diet eaten by most vegetarians can improve zinc status.

Zinc absorption is reduced by fiber, phytates, and calcium. According to the authors of the *Nutrition Desk Reference,* "Zinc absorption is impaired when large amounts of calcium in the diet bind with phytates and zinc in the intestine and form an insoluble complex."[56] Lacto-vegetarians, therefore, might want to offer their children dairy products independently of other zinc-rich foods.

Other Trace Minerals

The following minerals either are not usually lacking in a vegetarian diet or their role in human nutrition is not yet fully understood. The information presented below is primarily for interest rather than concern.

Arsenic's role in the human body is unclear, but it appears to be connected to the heart and skeletal muscles, methionine metabolism, the nervous and vascular systems, and blood clotting. Minute amounts of arsenic are found in water and in foods such as grains and starchy vegetables.

Boron may affect energy and mineral metabolism, including bone development and maintenance. Dietary boron mainly comes from water, fruits, vegetables, legumes, and nuts with much smaller amounts available from grains and dairy products.

Chromium is required for the synthesis of fatty acids, cholesterol and protein. It increases the effectiveness of insulin, and may improve immune function. Chromium is found in whole grains, legumes, nuts, seeds, fruits, vegetables, and brewer's yeast.

Cobalt is found in cobalamin. (*See vitamin B-12, page 77.*)

Nickel is used in enzymatic, hormonal, and cellular processes. Food sources of nickel include whole grains, legumes, nuts, and chocolate.

Silicon is found in connective tissues such as tendons, bones, and skin. Plants, especially whole grains, contain large amounts of silicon.

Vanadium deficiency has never been observed in humans, and its use in the body remains unknown. The ESADDI is approximately 100 micrograms/day, and it is available from foods such as mushrooms and parsley.

Other Nutritional Factors

Phytochemicals

"... [F]oods can no longer (and never could) be properly assessed only in terms of proteins, complex and simple carbohydrates, a few types of fat, a dozen vitamins, and fewer minerals. . . . vegetables and fruits . . . are chemical powerhouses that produce dozens if not hundreds of unique and complex organic compounds, many of which are biologically active . . . [and] may be able to affect significantly the quality and duration of life." [57]

Several different groups of beneficial phytochemicals have been identified. Bioflavinoids, for example, strengthen the immune and vascular systems, function as anti-oxidants, and may reduce the risk of developing cancer. Phenols, found abundantly in red wine, have been theorized to contribute to the prevention of certain chronic diseases. Phytosterols might protect the heart, and a number of other compounds (sulforaphane, ellagic acid, genistein) appear to inhibit the formation and progression of various cancers and other conditions.

Because phytochemicals are—by definition—found in plants (phyto means "plant," phytochemicals are literally "plant chemicals"), they are abundant in a whole food vegetarian diet. Especially phytochemical-rich foods to include in your family's diet are whole grains, legumes, soy products, nuts, seeds, cruciferous vegetables, tomatoes, garlic, leeks, onions, mushrooms, berries, red and black grapes, and citrus fruits, along with green tea for older children.

Some phytochemicals appear to act like estrogen in the body and so also are called phytoestrogens. The estrogenic activity of these substances is very mild compared to true estrogen and is thought to be a factor in the anti-cancer effects mentioned above. Questions have been raised, however, about the effect of phytoestrogens on the hormonal balance of infants. According to the authors of one study, there is ". . . little reason for concern . . . even when mothers consume soy during lactation. Because of the weak oestrogenic activity of isoflavones . . . the dietary intake of phyto-oestrogens from human milk is unlikely to exert biological effects." [58] As for soy formula, ". . . deleterious effects of soy-based infant formulas [have not] become apparent despite having been in use for more than 30 years . . . [but] long-term follow-up studies are needed to assess the potential beneficial or adverse effects of phyto-oestrogen exposure in early life." [59]

Fiber

Dietary fiber is a term that encompasses the parts of foods which are not digested but instead pass through the stomach and small intestines largely undisturbed (*see Simple and Complex Carbohydrates, page 67*). A combination of soluble and insoluble fiber can help remove certain undesirable substances from the body and is important for colonic health.[60] Fiber also helps the body determine when enough food has been eaten due to its bulking action in the stomach.

Infants naturally have a fiber-free diet for the first several months of life when breast milk (or formula) supplies them with a high-calorie, digestible food that will not strain their developing digestive system. As foods are added gradually during weaning, the fiber in the child's diet naturally will increase, thereby assisting your child to develop healthy eating patterns and proper bowel habits.

As your child begins to eat more fibrous foods, keep in mind that humans are designed to breast-feed for two or more years, so the high-fiber diet that might be appropriate for an adult could create problems for a young child. Not only can too much fiber displace the higher calorie foods a child needs, but fiber also is suspected of binding certain nutrients and preventing their complete absorption. By following the guidelines given in chapter six, you will learn how to supply your child with a diet that contains a good amount of fiber without displacing or interfering with the absorption of other, equally important nutrients.

Water

More than one hundred million Americans drink water that contains significant levels of three cancer-causing chemicals: arsenic, radon, and chlorine by-products (trihalomethanes, or THMs). Nitrates—which can cause deadly "blue-baby syndrome" when infant formula is made with tap water polluted by it—has [*sic*] been found at excessive levels in more than two thousand water systems in forty states. . . .

Andrew Weil, M.D.[61]

Water is obviously a vital dietary component, but under normal conditions your baby will not need to be given water while he or she is being exclusively breast- or bottle-fed, and probably not for some time into weaning.[62] However, offer water if the weather is unusually hot or your infant appears dehydrated. Your baby's pediatrician also may suggest water during periods of illness, especially when a fever is present.

When weaning is well under way, your child may express interest in water at which time it can be offered between meals. Remember that plant foods such as fruits and vegetables contain large amounts of water, and recommendations for water intake include the water found in food. As with any nutrient, too much water can create imbalances, both by depressing the appetite for nutritive foods, and by removing water-soluble nutrients from the body. Too little water, on the other hand, can contribute to constipation and dehydration. Teach your child about the importance of water, but allow your child to be the final judge of how much water he or she needs.

The most important thing you can do with regard to water is to make sure your water supply is safe. Both well water and tap water should be tested for dangerous substances such as nitrates, lead, and giardia. If you decide to install a filtration system, first find out what substances need to be filtered; then obtain the best quality system you can afford and maintain it regularly. A whole-house system is ideal as it removes substances like chlorine from bathing water as well as drinking water. At the very least, you probably will want an under-the-counter system that includes a KDF® filter followed by an activated carbon filter. Consumer guides can help you sort through the information in manufacturers' literature when making your purchase.

Finally, remember to ask your child's doctor about fluoride supplementation if your filter removes fluoride from the water.

RESOURCES

Don't Drink the Water: The Essential Guide to Our

Contaminated Drinking Water and What You Can Do About It by Lono Kahuna Kupua A'o (Kali Press, 1996)

Questions Concerning Eggs and Dairy Products

In 1997, the Vegetarian Resource Group sponsored a Roper Poll. The poll was well planned and executed, and the data obtained is considered to be some of the most accurate concerning the actual eating practices of vegetarians. Among the many interesting pieces of information gleaned from the poll was that "about one-third to one-half of the vegetarians appear to be vegans."[63]

Of course, this data implies that one-half to two-thirds of vegetarians still choose to eat dairy products and/or eggs. And if you are one of them, you might continue to want dairy products and eggs to be a part of your family's diet due to their familiarity and ease of preparation. Also, as the above discussion of nutrition shows, these animal products can supply important nutrients, such as vitamin B-12, calcium, and zinc, to your and your child's diet. But for all their strengths, eggs and dairy products are not necessarily benign foods, so if you are a lacto-ovo vegetarian parent, you should be aware of the possible pitfalls before deciding to feed them to your child.

Dairy products and eggs are animal products, and their negative nutritional qualities are much the same as those listed for meat at the beginning of this chapter—namely, cholesterol, saturated fat, lack of fiber, and potential contaminants.[64] Also, cheeses coagulated with rennet or milks supplemented with vitamin D derived from fish oils, are not, strictly speaking, vegetarian.

Even more troubling are specific problems related to use of these foods. Perhaps the best known is the tendency of dairy products to create allergies in susceptible children. Cows' milk is recognized as the number one cause of allergies and food sensitivities, affecting an estimated one to seven percent of children.[65-66] Many children (and their families) have found relief from chronic ear infections, constipation, and other allergy-related problems simply through the complete removal of dairy from the diet.[67]

And what about eggs? Eggs not only have extremely high levels of cholesterol and saturated fat, but they all too often carry food-poisoning organisms such as the Salmonella virus both outside and inside the shell. One study published in the *New England Journal of Medicine* stated that, "In the ten years from 1976 to 1986, the reported number of Salmonella enteritidis infections increased six-fold in the northeastern United States. [These] infections were specifically linked to consumption of foods containing eggs."[68]

If you do decide to continue using dairy products and eggs, and plan to give them to your child, you might want to search out local suppliers who have verifiably free-ranging, organically fed animals, who practice excellent hygiene, who make aged cheeses with vegetable rennet, and who use yeast-derived vitamin D-2 supplements in their milk. You also will want to read the information in chapter five about how to handle animal products correctly so as to avoid bringing contaminants into your kitchen, especially since young children are extremely vulnerable to such organisms.

Additional information on this topic is available from books which describe agribusiness operations. The titles listed below can help you gain a better understanding of the sanitation and health problems which are an inevitable result of large-scale factory farming. For more information on the nutritional aspects of eggs and dairy products, refer to the list of nutrition titles at the end of the chapter.

RESOURCES

Vegan: The New Ethics of Eating by Erik Marcus, McBooks Press, 1998.

Animal Factories by Jim Mason and Peter Singer, Harmony Books, 1990.

Prisoned Chickens Poisoned Eggs: An Inside Look at the Modern Poultry Industry by Karen Davis, Ph.D., Book Publishing Company, 1996.

Slaughterhouse: The Shocking Story of Greed, Neglect, and Inhumane Treatment Inside the U.S. Meat Industry by Gail A. Eisnitz, Prometheus Books, 1997.

Supplements and Fortified Foods

". . . [A] properly designed vegan diet should require no vitamin supplements, save B-12. Unless you have an unusual metabolism, vitamin supplements probably aren't needed except as a cheap nutritional insurance."

William Harris, M.D.[69]

Supplementation is always inferior to obtaining nutrients from foods. Nutrients don't exist in a vacuum, and taking single doses of any one nutrient can interfere with the absorption or utilization of others. Nutrition science also is not fully developed, and nutrition researchers continue to discover the importance of previously discounted nutrients (e.g., fiber, essential fatty acids) and to detect new substances (e.g., phytochemicals). By relying on a variety of whole foods to supply your family's nutrient needs, the possibility of missing an important, but as yet undiscovered, nutrient is reduced.

One reason to give your child supplements or fortified foods is that available natural sources of certain substances might, for some reason, be deficient. Three possible reasons for deficiency in plant foods that were identified above are location (iodine, selenium), season (vitamin D), and sanitation practices (vitamin B-12). Another reason is that when your child is growing fast, sometimes it can be difficult for him or her to eat enough to obtain everything that is needed (iron, calcium).

Your baby's pediatrician most likely will prescribe a child's multiple vitamin/mineral formulation just to make sure your child is getting the basics every day. Such formulations usually contain the DRI for most nutrients, including vitamin B-12, so additional supplementation generally is not necessary, especially for a child eating a whole foods diet.

If additional supplementation is desired, it is readily available in the form of fortified foods such as baby cereal (iron); soy, rice, or dairy milks (calcium, vitamin D, vitamin B-12); nutritional yeast (vitamin B-complex, vitamin B-12); fortified orange juice (calcium); and refined grain products (iron, vitamin B-complex, vitamin D). Nutrient-dense foods such as blackstrap molasses (iron, calcium) and flax seeds (omega-3 essential fatty acid) also can be used like supplements.

Care must be taken not to include so many supplements and fortified foods that your baby is harmed by an overdose. Many nutrients can safely be taken in relatively large quantities by adults, but babies are particularly vulnerable to excesses, and minerals and the fat-soluble vitamins especially should not be oversupplied. For example, fortification of cows' milk with vitamin D has been discontinued in Great Britain due to toxicity, and toxicity problems have occurred in the United States as well.[70] Another example is over-supplementation of fluoride leading to fluorosis.

Please note that many vitamin formulations contain substances that are derived from animal products. Vitamin D, for example, can be obtained from fish oil or lanolin (D-3) as well as yeast (D-2). Look for formulations that say "no animal products" or "vegetarian," and if you still are unsure, contact the company which makes the product. Finally, store the supplement in a dark, cool, dry place, and keep track of the expiration date.

Special note: Be absolutely sure to keep supplements out of the reach of your baby. Iron pills are the number one cause of poisoning deaths of children in America, and other supplements, like any concentrated product, also can endanger your child.[71]

Table 2.1

Recommendzed Dietary Allowances (RDA)[72]

	0 to 6 months (13 lbs., 24 oz.)*	6 to 12 months (20 lbs., 28 oz.)*	1 to 3 years (29 lbs., 35 oz.)*
Energy *(kcal)*	650	850	1300
Protein *(g)*	13	14	16
Vitamin A *(micrograms RE)*	375	375	400
Vitamin E *(milligrams α-TE)*	3	4	6
Vitamin K *(micrograms)*	5	10	15
Vitamin C *(milligrams)*	30	35	40
Iron *(milligrams)*	6	10	10
Zinc *(milligrams)*	5	5	10
Iodine *(micrograms)*	40	50	70
Selenium *(micrograms)*	10	15	20

Note: With few exceptions, breast milk from a well-nourished woman naturally supplies complete nutrition for infants and substantial nutrients for older babies and toddlers until they are weaned. Commercial infant formula is the only way to ensure proper nutrition for a bottle-fed infant.

* *A child weighing up to*

Table 2.2

Dietary Reference Intakes (DRI)[73]

	0 to 6 months (13 lbs., 24 oz.)*	6 to 12 months (20 lbs., 28 oz..)*	1 to 3 years (29 lbs., 35 oz.)*
Vitamin D (micrograms)	5	5	5
Vitamin B-1 (Thiamin) (milligrams)	0.2	0.3	0.5
Vitamin B-2 (Riboflavin) (milligrams)	0.3	0.4	0.5
Vitamin B-3 (Niacin) (milligrams NE)	2	4	6
Vitamin B-6 (Pyridoxine) (milligrams)	0.1	0.3	0.5
Pantothenic Acid (milligrams)	1.7	1.8	2
Choline (milligrams)	125	150	200
Biotin (micrograms)	5	6	8
Folate (micrograms)	65	80	150
Vitamin B-12 (micrograms)	0.4	0.5	0.9
Calcium (milligrams)	210	270	500
Fluoride (milligrams)	0.01	0.5	0.7
Phosphorus (milligrams)	100	275	460
Magnesium (milligrams)	30	75	80

Note: The values for infants are Adequate Intakes (AI) for healthy, breast-fed infants. The values for toddlers are either AIs or RDAs. DRIs presently are being developed for the nutrients not listed in this table. Until the new data are released, the RDAs in Table 2.1 should be used.

* A child weighing up to

Table 2.3

Essential and Semi-essential Amino Acids in Selected Foods[74]

Grams of amino acid per 100 grams edible portion

	Kale (boiled)	Kidney Beans (boiled)	Oatmeal (cooked)	Almond Butter	Cows' Milk	Human Milk	Egg
Isoleucine	0.1	0.4	0.1	0.7	0.2	0.10	0.7
Leucine	0.1	0.7	0.2	1.2	0.3	0.10	1.1
Lysine	0.1	0.6	0.1	0.5	0.3	0.10	0.8
Threonine	0.1	0.4	0.1	0.6	0.1	0.04	0.6
Tryptophan	0.02	0.1	0.04	0.3	0.05	0.02	0.2
Valine	0.1	0.5	0.1	0.8	0.2	0.10	0.9
Methionine	0.02	0.1	0.05	0.2	0.1	0.02	0.4
Phenylalanine	0.1	0.5	0.1	0.8	0.2	0.05	0.7
Arginine	0.1	0.5	0.2	1.9	0.1	0.04	0.8
Histidine	0.04	0.2	0.1	0.4	0.1	0.02	0.3

RESOURCES

Vegan Nutrition by Gil Langley (Vegan Society, 1995).

Becoming Vegetarian: The Complete Guide to Adopting a Healthy Vegetarian Diet by Vesanto Melina, Brenda Davis, and Victoria Harrison (Book Publishing Company, 1995).

The Dietitian's Guide to Vegetarian Diets: Issues and Applications by Mark Messina and Virginia Messina (Aspen Publishers, 1996).

The Vegetarian Way: Total Health for You and Your Family by Virginia Messina and Mark Messina (Three Rivers Press, 1996).

Pediatric Nutrition Handbook, Fourth Edition, edited by Ronald E. Kleinman, (The Committee on Nutrition, American Academy of Pediatrics, 1998).

Dr. Spock's Baby and Child Care by Benjamin Spock and Steven J. Parker (Simon & Schuster, 1998).

The Yale Guide to Children's Nutrition edited by William V. Tamborlane (Yale University Press, 1997).

THREE

Vegetarian Parents

When we change the way we grow our food, we change our food, we change society, we change our values. And so this book is about paying attention to relationships, to causes and effects and it is about being responsible for what one knows . . . we cannot isolate one aspect of life from another.

Wendell Berry[1]

Pregnancy

SHARON'S STORY: *Before Birth*

I have been a "mostly" vegetarian for about ten years—the "mostly" referring to occasional seafood and chicken included in my diet throughout. However, the father of my baby is a much stricter vegetarian; he eats no meat, although he occasionally eats . . . dairy products. While I was pregnant, we mutually decided that we both believed in vegetarianism as a way of life and would raise our child in that way. At the time of the decision, it seemed unreal that I would ever have an actual baby in my arms to whom I would offer a vegetarian diet.

• • •

 IT IS VERY important to be aware of nutrition while you are pregnant, and to get into the habit of eating well. The requirements for all nutrients do increase during pregnancy; the answer, however, is not to eat meat, but to start eating a high-quality, nutrient-dense diet early in pregnancy, or even before conception. This chapter provides a very complete answer to the question, "Is it safe to be a vegetarian/vegan while I am pregnant?" Taking care of yourself is the first way you can show love for your baby. Avoiding meats and the chemicals involved in their production, eschewing over-processed and under-nutritious foods, and avoiding drugs and other non-food chemicals will give your baby a much healthier start. Good health for babies, in other words, begins before birth.

Although the father's role before birth affects a child less on the strictly physical level, his support is important to a mother's well-being, if he is to be involved at all. A father who takes special care to eat well, and who prepares nutritious, tasty meals for the mother during pregnancy, is helping to create a healthy baby almost as certainly as she does in actually transferring the nutrients to the unborn child. Pregnancy, and nutrition during pregnancy, should be a cooperative venture.

Nutrition Guidelines

The following nutrients are those which vegetarian women are advised to be especially aware of during pregnancy. Each nutrient is discussed in detail in chapter two; the additional information provided here is specific to the needs of mothers. As you read, you are encouraged to refer back to the related entries in chapter two for more details about each nutrient, including lists of dietary sources.

The numbers given with each entry are the RDAs and DRIs for pregnancy. A complete listing of the dietary recommendations for pregnant and lactating women are available in Tables 3.1 and 3.2, and a "Vegetarian Food Guide for Pregnant and Lactating Women" is included at the end of this section, as well. Pregnancy is not the focus of this book, however. For much more detailed information, the following books are recommended.

Vegetarian Pregnancy by Sharon Yntema (McBooks Press, 1994).

Pregnancy, Children, and the Vegan Diet by Michael Klaper, MD (Gentle World, 1988).

ENERGY AND WEIGHT GAIN

RDA for energy during pregnancy: normal intake +300 kcal/day

General guidelines for pregnancy are the same for vegetarian women as they are for omnivores. You, therefore, should strive to eat enough energy-dense food to gain weight according to standard charts, as your baby needs the energy to grow, and along with the extra calories come the extra nutrients you both need, so long as you choose healthful foods. Most women should seek to gain 25 to 35 pounds, but very thin women should try to gain more (28 to 40 pounds), and overweight women can usually gain less (15 to 25 pounds). Teenagers and women carrying multiple fetuses have special requirements that are best met with a larger than normal weight gain (30 to 45 pounds and 35 to 45 pounds, respectively).

PROTEIN

RDA for protein during pregnancy: 60 g/day

Protein needs increase by 15 to 25 percent during pregnancy. This extra protein is needed for the growth of the fetus and placenta as well as the mother's expanding uterus, enlarging breasts, and increasing blood volume. The addition of an extra serving every day of concentrated protein foods such as legumes, seitan, soy products, high-protein grains (quinoa, amaranth), dairy products, and eggs should easily cover your increased needs. Legume-based puréed soups, tofu, soy or dairy milks and yogurts, and eggs are especially good foods at this time as liquids and bland foods can be easier to digest through bouts of morning sickness and as your stomach is compressed during the latter months of pregnancy. A serving of soy or rice-based protein powder also can be added to other foods if your appetite is so poor that you have trouble eating enough high-protein foods.

FAT

RDA for fat during pregnancy: none established

A small increase in the amount of fat you eat is an easy way to meet your increased energy needs. The quality of the fats you choose is very important as undesirable chemicals can concentrate in fat tissues, and you won't want to pass those on to your developing baby. If you possibly can, buy fresh, organically grown nuts, seeds and oils. If you choose to use eggs and dairy products, make sure they are hormone-free and that the animals are fed organic feed.

You should be sure to include some fatty foods that are rich in omega-3 essential fatty acids (EFAs), which your baby needs for proper nervous system development. You need not overeat fats to meet this requirement. A few teaspoons of flaxseed oil (excellent on toast or in a salad dressing), or a meal with leafy greens, walnuts, and tofu, contain a plentiful amount of omega-3s. You should also follow other good nutritional principles such as avoiding saturated and trans fats, and emphasizing whole foods such as avocados and seeds.

Some concern has been expressed regarding the ability of vegans to convert the EFAs to other "long-chain," non-essential fatty acids, especially docosahexanoic acid (DHA). In a study of the fatty acid profile of human breast milk, both vegan and lacto-ovo vegetarians produced milk with more EFAs than that of omnivorous women, but vegans were found to have half as much DHA in their milk as both lacto-ovo vegetarians and omnivores.[2] Until more information is available, you might ask your doctor about taking a DHA supplement throughout pregnancy and lactation, especially if you eat a vegan diet. Unfortunately, most such supplements aren't vegetarian; one which is (Neuromins), presently is packaged in gelatin (non-vegetarian) capsules.

Infant formula is expected to be fortified with EFAs and DHA, in the near future. Vegetarian parents can increase the demand for plant-derived sources of these nutrients by contacting formula and supplement manufacturers.[3-4]

FOLATE

DRI for folate during pregnancy: 600 micrograms DFE/day

All the vitamins are important for proper fetal development, but supplemental folate in particular has been identified as preventing neural tube birth defects when taken before conception and through the early months of pregnancy.

A list of foods rich in B vitamins, including folate, is given under the vitamin B-complex entry in chapter two. Vegetarian diets usually supply a generous amount of folate unless the diet is inconsistent or contains few vegetables or a large amount of processed foods. Even if you eat an excellent diet, however, a pre-conception and then a pre-natal supplement that contain the water-soluble B vitamins certainly will not hurt you and can give you and your loved ones peace of mind. Don't take more than the recommended amount of supplemental folate as it can interfere with absorption of other nutrients such as zinc and iron.

VITAMIN B-12

DRI for vitamin B-12 during pregnancy: 2.6 micrograms/day

Vitamin B-12 is discussed in detail in chapter two. Vegans, and lacto-ovo vegetarians who eat few eggs or dairy products, will definitely want to make sure to include a reliable source of vitamin B-12 daily throughout pregnancy. This vitamin is needed for blood formation and during times of rapid growth, so it is vital to the healthy development of the fetus.

VITAMIN D

DRI for vitamin D during pregnancy: 5 micrograms/day

Vitamin D is essential for proper development of your baby's skeleton, and a fetus can develop skeletal problems such as rickets even when the mother shows no overt sign of deficiency. So, even though your own body certainly can produce ample vitamin D if exposed to enough spring and summer sunlight, you definitely will want to take supplemental vitamin D during pregnancy if it is winter or if your time in the sun is at all limited. A prenatal supplement should contain the DRI for vitamin D, and vitamin D also is available from fortified foods, but remember not to overdo supplemental sources of this fat-soluble and potentially toxic vitamin.

CALCIUM

DRI for calcium during pregnancy: 1000 milligrams/day

While pregnant, you must meet your baby's substantial calcium needs along with your own. Lacto-vegetarians generally can meet the increased need for calcium by eating several servings of dairy products each day. That much dairy is not necessarily benign, however (*see Questions Concerning Eggs and Dairy Products page 95*), so please note that it is possible to meet calcium needs through use of calcium-rich plant foods such as kale, sea vegetables, and tahini, along with fortified foods such as fortified soy milk and fortified orange juice. Strive to eat several servings a day of these foods, and ask your doctor about calcium supplementation if your appetite is depressed. Though calcium is important, eating more than the DRI is not advisable because it can create imbalances in other nutrients.

IRON

RDA for iron during pregnancy: 30 milligrams/day

The RDA for iron during pregnancy is so high it is difficult to obtain from food alone, even for omnivores. A pre-natal supplement will contain plentiful iron. Some women find supplemental iron to cause problems such as constipation, however, so if you prefer to obtain your nutrients from your diet, strive to eat as many iron-rich foods as you can, especially concentrated ones such as blackstrap molasses and dried figs. You also can increase your iron absorption by cooking as many meals as possible in cast-iron pans, adding side dishes which contain raw, vitamin C-rich fruits and vegetables, and eating any dairy products separately from iron-rich foods.

ZINC

RDA for zinc during pregnancy: 15 milligrams/day

Zinc is usually listed as a nutrient of concern for vegetarians, especially during pregnancy, because zinc tends to be less available from plants. Be sure to include zinc-rich foods in your diet, and try to eat them separately from calcium-rich foods such as dairy products. And, of course, a pre-natal supplement or fortified foods can help you meet your zinc requirement if diet alone is not enough.

Herbal Preparations

Many health-conscious people have elected to include herbs in their diets both for nutritive and medicinal purposes. Some herbs are neutral or beneficial, but others can be harmful—and possibly even fatal—to your fetus.[5] This is obvious if you stop to think that any substance powerful enough to create noticeable effects in the adult body could potentially have an extreme effect on your fetus or child, especially if poorly manufactured or used improperly. For example, a recent issue of the *New England Journal of Medicine* contains reports of problems such as lead poisoning, nausea, diarrhea, and abnormal heart rhythms resulting from the use of herbs and other "natural, drug-free" products.[6]

The American Academy of Pediatrics recommends limiting herbal teas to 16 ounces per day. Safe herbal teas include mint and rosehip, as well as fruit teas such as lemon and red raspberry. If you consult an herbalist, make sure he or she is well trained, reputable, and uses only the highest quality products. And you should, of course, discuss any use of herbs with your doctor before you take them, and carefully monitor any reactions.

Natural Baby Care: Pure and Soothing Recipes and Techniques for Mothers and Babies by Colleen K. Dodt (Storey Communications, 1997).

Wise Woman Herbal for the Childbearing Years by Susan Weed, (Ash Tree Publishing, 1986).

Lactation

The milk of vegetarian mothers is nutritionally adequate, and breast-fed infants of well-nourished vegetarian women grow and develop normally.

The Dietitian's Guide to Vegetarian Diets[7]

Unless bottle-fed, newborns are completely dependent on mother's milk for the first months of life, so the special care that a mother gives herself and her developing child during pregnancy should not stop upon birth. The diet that was eaten by the mother during pregnancy should be continued through the months of lactation, but the proportions of many nutrients are changed. For example, the Recommended Dietary Allowance for energy increases significantly during lactation. Vitamin A requirements also rise, as do protein needs, and vitamin C, riboflavin, iodine, and zinc requirements. On the other hand, iron and folic acid requirements drop substantially. (*See Tables 3.1 and 3.2, pages 133 and 134, for details.*)

As for supplements, notice that requirements for almost all nutrients remain higher than for the non-pregnant, non-lactating woman, so a multi-vitamin/mineral or fortified foods can continue to help meet those increased needs. Supplemental vitamin B-12 continues to be necessary for vegan and near-vegan mothers as it must be present in the diet in order for enough to be incorporated into breast milk. Vitamins A, B-complex, C, and D, fatty acids, and possibly some minerals also will vary in the breast milk according to the mother's diet.

Contaminants

In an analysis of [chemicals in] breast milk . . . the highest vegan value was lower than the lowest value seen in breast milk samples from the general population. In most cases, levels were only 1 percent to 2 percent of those in the samples from the general population.[8]

There have been some scares about the pesticide content of nursing mothers' milk. According to the authors of one research study, ". . . many chemicals have been detected in breast milk in recent years. As a principle, each substance that is not naturally present in breast milk or whose concentrations are above normal levels is considered a contaminant These substances cause concerns regarding the health of the newborn who is exclusively fed with this nutrition."[9]

Many common sense health practices can help protect against such contamination. Obviously, as much of your diet as possible should be from organically grown sources, especially with regards to animal products and high-fat plant foods since contaminants often concentrate in fatty tissues. Washing all produce in water—even produce that is organically grown—can reduce or remove many contaminants. Produce soaps are not necessary, but if you use them make sure to rinse the produce especially well. You also can peel produce, but the peels of many fruits and vegetables contain nutrients you won't want to discard so that is not an optimal solution. Drinking and cooking with filtered water is a good idea, as is avoiding toxic chemicals at home and at work.

Many vegetarians follow these guidelines which probably accounts for the fact that the breast milk of vegetarians tends to contain substantially fewer contaminants than that of omnivores. No place on our polluted planet is completely free of contamination, so just do the best you can with the tools at your disposal.

General Health

In addition to maintaining a healthy diet, drink lots of liquid (you may notice you get very thirsty whenever you nurse—pay attention to your body!). Mild exercise and relaxation techniques such as meditation, visualization, and deep breathing, are tremendously helpful. You also should get as much rest and sleep as possible, although that is extremely difficult with an infant in the house. If you can, lie down when you nurse, and ask your friends and family members for help so you don't become overextended.

Support groups can offer more specific and personal advice than can fit into any book. Ask your doctor how to get in touch with a group in your town, or contact one of the organizations listed below. The emotional support alone makes such groups worthwhile, especially during the first few weeks after birth when physical exhaustion and emotional letdown can lead to depression and anxiety.

Finally, talk to other parents, vegetarian or not, for special tips and the wisdom of personal experience. Rest, eat well, love yourself, and enjoy your baby!

RESOURCES

The Womanly Art of Breast-feeding by La Leche League (Penguin Putnam, 1997).

La Leche League International, Inc.
1400 N. Meacham Rd., Schaumburg, IL 60173-4048
847-519-7730; http://www.lalecheleague.org

International Childbirth Education Association
P.O. Box 20048; Minneapolis, MN 55420
612-854-8660; http://www.icea.org

Weaning

SHARON'S STORY: *From Breast to Bottle to Cup*

When my son was eight and a half months old, I developed an infection which was serious enough to require a very heavy dose of Flagyl, a drug which contaminates breast milk and is not good for the baby. I was abruptly forced to stop nursing for two weeks, which gave me a much more sympathetic understanding of mothers who are unable to nurse. It was probably more traumatic for me than for my baby. He took to a bottle of goats' milk and yogurt (mixed and strained to remove the lumps) very willingly, although he was certainly confused by the change. I expressed milk during the two weeks and then started nursing him again. I decided, however, to continue the bottle partially, because it meant my husband had more of a chance to feed our baby, which was an important sharing experience.

I have found that even though I welcome the switch to feeding my son adult meals, I feel nostalgic at times for the early nursing moments, for his first taste of yogurt, and for the sour faces he made when tasting a new food which he always followed by reaching for more of the same food. The lesson that I have learned through watching my son grow is that each moment is special, even if it is filled with frustration, and especially when it is filled with his smiles.

• • •

Whether weaning means the introduction of a bottle and/or solid foods, or the end of nursing altogether, a change from an all-milk diet is a very important time for both parent and child. Suddenly, the ease of knowing that all the nutrients are supplied in the correct amounts is gone and must be replaced by a conscious decision about what to feed the baby, while making sure he or she continues to be healthy.

Most experts agree that nursing should continue for a minimum of six months, and preferably for one to two years. By extending the period of nursing for as long as possible (from two up to five years), you will continue to supply important nutrients to your child's diet, even after weaning is well underway. You child also will appreciate the added comfort and emotional bonding that occurs with prolonged nursing.

As your child's intake of breast milk decreases, you can gradually shift back to your pre-pregnancy diet and activities. Allow the responses of your child and your own body, as well as your personal needs, to guide you in making this shift.

For the vegetarian parent, weaning is often an especially exciting event as it means not just that your child is growing, but that you can begin to share the important world view exemplified by your diet. The mechanics of the weaning process are described in chapters four and six, but you undoubtedly will find the reality to be an incredible time of alternating challenges and delight!

Managing Home and Work

SHARON'S STORY: *Back to the Office*

When my baby was one month old, I returned to work on a part-time basis. I worked three evenings a week while my husband took care of the baby. Although it was new and hard for him, I think my absence gave him a special early relationship with our baby that many men do not have a chance to experience. I was able to express several ounces of milk for each evening I was away. If this ran out, my husband fed him a yogurt and water mixture.

When my baby was five months old, I started to work during the day so that it was no longer possible to leave him with his father. Fortunately, I was able to find a very good situation in which the caregivers appreciated and accepted my vegetarian feeding ideas as they applied to my son, who was beginning to eat solid foods.

However, working more hours (five mornings a week) cut severely into my free time, and I found that it was difficult to spend a great deal of time making meals for my son. I developed the casserole idea and the fine grinding of grains which, in effect, produced "instant meals," both of which are described in detail later in this book. I didn't freeze foods, finding it quicker (or at least as quick) to prepare small amounts from fresh foods than to thaw out frozen portions. I developed a pattern of feeding my son first and then giving him foods he could pick up with his fingers as we ate, so that we could share our mealtimes without my food getting cold as I fed him.

I have found in general that feeding a baby is an exciting and painless activity, despite the time pressure my job added to my daily life as a mother. (Fortunately, my husband and I have always shared the making of meals, so that even though he worked all day outside the house while I only worked half a day, we took turns getting our meals ready rather than my having to have a meal on the table when he got home from work.) I have found that, although I am not an avid cook, I have really enjoyed preparing foods for my baby. He is willing to try anything once, as the saying goes.

Even though working can add pressure to a family's life, it is possible to make mealtime a relaxed, sharing, and enjoyable time. I never eat frozen prepared foods, and the short cuts I take do not cut nutritional corners, but only time.

· · ·

Being a working parent should not have to mean that non-working time becomes rushed with a young child. It is possible to remain calm and healthy while working both inside and outside the home. This is a good thing as most people in our society do combine paid employment and family life. According to the United States Department of Health and Human Services, "In 1995, about 62 percent of all mothers with preschool-aged children (younger than six years) were in the labor force, a nearly twofold increase since 1970."[10] This statistic translates into about 10 million women and 12 million children.[11] Given that fathers have traditionally worked outside the home, what this means is that the vast majority of parents work while simultaneously raising their children. In other words, you are not alone.

All of those families are generating a fundamental change in our society. Many fathers are becoming more involved with the day-to-day care of their children. Quality child care services are easier to come by, and progressive businesses are providing maternity and paternity leave, day care, and other child-related services for employees. A large variety of convenience foods, including healthy vegetarian ones, and time-saving kitchen appliances, help ease the transition as well.

Nursing, and the desire to provide a vegetarian diet for your youngster, do complicate matters, so you will need to figure out how to feed your child when he or she is in the care of others.

Many parents have found creative solutions through the manipulation of their child's eating schedule, changes in their own work schedules, and the use of expressed milk fed from a bottle. Upon weaning, they then learn to prepare fast foods that can be easily transported and stored, and which don't make their children feel too "different" in the company of peers. Chapters five and six offer some ideas for such quick and easy meal preparation.

No matter what your diet, one tactic for efficient and blame-free family management is to design an explicit "parenting contract" which outlines each family member's duties regarding child care, household management, and joint public and social life. An article by Anne Chappell Belden which appeared in the Summer/Fall 1998 issue of the *San Francisco Bay Area Baby Resource Guide,* outlines just such a contract. She suggests deciding before the birth who will send out announcements, bathe the baby, do the dishes, pay the bills, and stay home when the baby is ill. Her contract even includes space to schedule some time for parents to be alone together, and to figure out who will be responsible for finding a baby-sitter and planning the occasion. You also can add sections concerning parenting goals and values which can help alleviate friction down the line.

Other lactating mothers and vegetarian parents can give you practical advice and emotional support, so joining a parenting group or local vegetarian organization is a good idea. The time you give to such groups will be amply repaid by the information and care you receive in return, especially if your group is willing to rotate child care and shopping duties over the course of the week, leaving you free to concentrate on your work on the days you are not "it." This will be easier if the other parents also are vegetarian, but that is not mandatory so long as your requirements regarding your child and your own participation are clear.

RESOURCES

Nursing Mother, Working Mother: The Essential Guide for Breast-feeding and Staying Close to Your Baby After You Return to Work by Gale Pryor (Harvard Common Press, 1997)

Breast-feeding and the Working Mother by Diane Mason (St. Martin's Press, 1997)

Caring For Your Baby and Young Child: Birth to Age 5 by the American Academy of Pediatricians (American Academy of Pediatrics, 1998). Chapters 14 and 22 are especially helpful.

Interacting with Others

Inevitably, there will be times when you will be called upon to explain—or even justify—your child's diet to others. These can be family members concerned about your child's health, a doctor who insists you feed your child meat or dairy products, day care workers who express concern over your child's physical and social development, or strangers in the line at the grocery store checkout. It pays to be prepared for such interactions.

The first thing you must determine upon being asked questions is whether the questioner has a right or need to know such details about your family. Vegetarian parents often are justifiably proud of their child's diet and want to talk about it to everyone they meet. For the safety of your child, you should consider curbing this impulse. Most people do not encounter problems, but some have had experiences you would not want to repeat. One father, for example, had to fight the state of California to regain custody of his daughter after she was removed from his care due to a misunderstanding by the school nurse of both the girl's vegetarian diet and her congenital health problems.[12] Another family lost the child they had adopted after the adoption agency found out they were raising him as a vegetarian.[13-14] Divorce proceedings are another time when a vegetarian parent can face discrimination. This doesn't mean you should live in fear, but it is a good idea to exercise prudence when speaking to others. If someone who has no right to know is asking questions, all you need say is, "We prefer not to discuss our family's diet."

If you have determined that someone has a legitimate reason to know about your child's diet, you will be much more convincing if you are well educated and informed on the subject. Reading this book is a good first step, but you might consider educating yourself further about vegetarian nutrition for children by reading some of the reference books listed at the end of chapter two and in the bibliography. Joining a reputable organization such as the Vegetarian Resource Group, or contacting a local dietitian who belongs to the American Dietetic Association's Vegetarian Practice Group (DPG #14), are other ways of keeping up to date. You then will have access to convincing materials to give to skeptics.

You also will want to keep good records, especially if your child tends toward the small side or suffers from some illness or problem that affects growth or learning ability. People who are prejudiced against vegetarianism will blame such problems on diet without thinking how silly it is to assume a few bites of meat or sips of cows' milk would cause the child from a naturally small-statured family to grow to a great size, or would miraculously cure something such as fetal alcohol syndrome or a congenital neurological disorder. By keeping track of your child's diet, medical, and family history, you will have the information you need to answer questions if they should arise.

Finally, be firm. You have taken the time to read this book and to learn how to feed your child a healthy vegetarian diet. If you know that your child is thriving, mentally and physically, then others will not be able to intimidate you, and you can answer legitimate questions with confidence.

Interviews with Vegetarian Parents

SHARON'S STORY: *Sharing with Others*

The information that I read concerning the nutrition of pregnant and nursing mothers sometimes seemed too impersonal, even though I knew it was a very essential part of raising a vegetarian baby. I felt that I understood this information much more clearly when I talked with other parents who already had a baby or babies and who were raising healthy vegetarian children. Every parent had a unique story to share.

• • •

It is hard to write a book that will answer all the questions anyone could ask about raising a vegetarian baby. The scope of this book, therefore, has been broadened by including comments from vegetarian parents. Their varied insights, experiences, and lifestyles add depth to the subject of raising children as vegetarians.

Interviews

The first transcript is from Sharon Yntema's own journal, an "interview" with herself which traces her son's development through a nine-month period at the beginning of his life (he is now an adult). It is followed by excerpts from reports graciously provided by a number of other vegetarian parents who currently are raising vegetarian children. Out of the 48 families who responded to a call for interviews, 25 returned a questionnaire, with 12 providing more detailed information. Although by no means a scientific survey, the information and stories that have been offered paint an intriguing picture of vegetarianism in this country during the latter part of the twentieth century.

Sharon; baby Nikolas (New York)

"Five months: I feel very ambivalent about starting solid foods with Nikolas. On the one hand, I am excited to be able to try out all the recipes I can think of and to watch his delighted (or not so delighted) expressions as I give him the very little tastes of what I am eating. However, I am nervous about changing from a complete nursing-milk diet in which I know he is getting all the vitamins, minerals and proteins he needs. How can I be sure he is getting everything he needs without consulting a food composition chart as I cook each food?

"Six months: I am still relying greatly on nursing for Nikolas to get the nutrients he needs. I am introducing foods now, mostly to see what he thinks of the taste. He seems to like everything I give him and goes 'eh-eh-eh' for more. Sometimes he tries to hold the spoon after he has eaten a little from it. The rest somehow ends up on the back of his head. So far he has tasted yogurt, apple juice, orange juice, prune juice, nectarines, oatmeal, rice, bananas, peaches, and avocados.

"Seven months: It's hard to make sure he gets enough vegetables in his diet—especially the stronger-tasting ones like broccoli. I still worry that he's not getting enough of everything and feel relieved only because he is still nursing. The pediatrician says not to worry about the amount of iron he's getting, although everything I read seems to say that a baby's iron stores run out between four to six months. I try to combine orange juice and eggs (the vitamin C in the orange juice assists iron absorption from the eggs) to make sure, though. I tried giving Nikolas some of the packaged iron-fortified baby cereal—he grimaced and spit it out. No wonder! I tried it and it tasted like gummy cardboard. Usually I really like everything I make for him, although I tend to want to salt it for myself. I'm using kelp instead of salt for Nikolas to make sure that he is getting enough iodine.

"Seven and one-half months—a typical day's menu:

Breakfast: cereal with banana and yogurt

Snack: apple juice

Lunch: cottage cheese and applesauce with ground-up wheat germ

Snack: nursing

Dinner: grain and vegetable with yogurt (or egg and vegetable, or tofu and grain and vegetable); juice to drink

Bedtime: nursing

All night and first thing in the morning: nursing

"Eight months: Foods that he has tried so far (I haven't been as careful about allergies as the books say to, partly because I figure I started feeding him pretty late, so that allergies are less likely to happen): yogurt, cottage cheese, banana, apple, pears, mango, papaya, avocado, peaches, figs, prune juice, orange juice, carrots, yellow squash, zucchini, green beans, peas, corn, lima beans, rice (brown rice), millet, barley, oatmeal, tofu, egg yolk, wheat germ, coconut (juice and meat), lentils.

"Eight and one-half months: I have to stop nursing because of medication that I have to take. How will he survive without the 'perfect' diet?

"Nine months: Nikolas seems to eat really well when there are other children around—partly he is so entranced by watching them that I'm not sure he is aware that he is eating.

"Ten months: I'm back to nursing but my milk supply seems low—I rarely hear him swallow a lot. He wants to eat by himself these days—he bats away a spoon most of the time but will feed himself dozens of peas and pieces of cheese, crackers, and lentils. Lentils, in fact, are really a favorite, especially my casserole which has wheat germ, lentils, garlic, onions, and egg in it. He loves scrambled eggs made with milk, but spits them out when they are made without milk. He has the most incredible expressions of distaste and even pretends to gag when he doesn't want to eat something—I say 'pretends' because sometimes he gags before the food even gets to his mouth, and he always smiles or laughs after he gags, in a very knowing way.

"Ten and one-half months: He doesn't seem to be eating much of anything, but seems to want to nurse, nurse, nurse, about 85 times a day. He won't eat chunks of food that he used to love; won't eat from a spoon (more than a couple of bites), won't drink more than a couple of ounces from a bottle. He doesn't seem to get frustrated that there is little milk in my breasts, but will suck endlessly.

"I've been trying different techniques to get him to eat other than nursing. One of the most effective is feeding him in the bathtub while he plays in the water; he'll eat tremendous amounts while he's doing something else. From what I've heard and read this is a common stage, and it is better to have the child enjoy eating even if it means playing at the same time than to force him and set up a bad feeling about food. Nikolas just seems to dislike a formal mealtime, no matter how much fun I try to make it.

"Eleven and one-half months: Nikolas has started enjoying mealtimes again and can eat tremendous amounts—practically twice as much as he did a month ago. He doesn't seem to want to feed himself with a spoon, although he likes to drink from a cup, holding it himself. I try to give him something that he can pick up with his fingers and eat at each meal, because he seems to enjoy that. I usually feed him first and then give him bits and pieces of whatever I'm eating, when I eat. He doesn't like peas now—if I give him a spoonful of mushed grains or yogurt with a whole pea, he will eat the food and casually spit out the pea when he's done—it must take a lot of control not to mash it up as he moves his mouth around the other food! Although I am still nursing, Nikolas drinks six to eight ounces of milk from a bottle during the afternoon and before his bedtime. The nursing seems to have a last relaxing effect so that he can conk out at night. I've added broccoli and cabbage to his regular vegetables, in combination with grains, and he likes them fine. He still goes through periods of not eating well during one meal, but then eating well the next one. He definitely lets me know when he is through eating: he shakes his head and pushes my hands away—no question about overstuffing him or forcing him to eat. He doesn't seem to like breads and crackers as much as he used to, but loves cheese. When he eats yogurt, he looks like a TV commercial for a yogurt company—eating with such eagerness and perfect form. A nonparent friend of mine has asked me if I have to think about what I'm going to feed him next, sounding like it was a burden. I do have to think, but I feel like I'm able to create the most wonderful gourmet dishes for my special baby.

"One year: Nikolas is learning to share. He gives me his food to eat and wants to eat mine. I like it better, though, when he shares his orange juice popsicle than when he tries to share his baby mush. It's a nice thought, though!

"Fourteen months: Nikolas is feeding himself very well these days, so I give him a thick mush food as a main meal most of the time. He uses a spoon, although he turns it over right before it gets to his mouth, so that if the meal is too runny, he loses half of it. He can hold a cup alone although he still tends to spill it when he is distracted by anything. He signals to me when he is through eating by dropping his spoon and bowl over the edge of the table, unless I am quick enough to catch it first."

Christine and Kyle; baby Meara (Michigan)

Meara was born in 1996 and is being weaned to a vegan diet by her parents, Christine and Kyle, who have been vegetarian since 1993 and vegan since 1996. Christine writes:

"People who don't know Meara is vegan are always commenting on how well she eats vegetables. Her favorites are beets, carrots, olives, pickles, cucumbers, and broccoli. She goes right for the veggie plate at a party. On the other hand, she doesn't really notice wrapped candy as something to eat. She will play with it, but not really eat it. As for nursing, we did the whole La Leche family-bed thing with no problems. We are now starting to nurse very infrequently during the day, and Meara sleeps part of the night in her own bed, so we nurse less at night, too.

"Meara has had three ear infections. We gave her antibiotics the first time, but when we switched doctors, we found one who monitors rather than prescribes antibiotics. She's also had a few colds, a couple of fevers, chicken pox, and, we think, roseola. She's had all the same sicknesses as all the kids around here. She is normal in size, bouncing from the 75th to 90th percentiles in height and weight. She tends to be taller than average and has lots of baby fat (although she really slimmed down when she started to walk).

"I sought out doctors who are sympathetic, but [I] have had a lot of problems with family. When my husband's family found out, they threatened to cancel Thanksgiving even though we were supposed to be in labor that day and so wouldn't have been at the get-together anyway. My mother wants to be supportive, but my father and stepmother pretty much avoid us. I guess it is hard on everyone because they can't give my daughter all the goodies they want to, like ice cream. Their attitude that we shouldn't inconvenience them for her health irritates me, but I find I can bear it by just repeating my stand.

"My sister cares for Meara, and as far as I can tell, respects our diet. I provide a packed lunch each day she goes to her aunt's. I've been so concerned about finding vegan-friendly day care when

I go back to work full-time that I've even considered starting one. I also might home-school, if necessary. Our playgroup is relatively supportive. If Meara dips her chip in a dairy-based dip, I just replace it with a vegan alternative and repeat our dietary stance nicely."

Teresa; baby Tara Rose (Washington)

Tara Rose has a vegetarian mother and a non-vegetarian father. She will be weaned onto a vegan diet. Writes Teresa:

"I had been a vegetarian for ten years and [had been] moving towards a vegan diet for about 12 months, when I discovered I was pregnant in the fall of 1997. Many of my friends were concerned about my vegetarian diet and tried to persuade me to eat meat. I decided to join a vegetarian organization for social support. The group I joined has many active members and a monthly vegan potluck. Talking with other vegetarian parents gave me the support and humor I needed both during and after the pregnancy.

"Tara Rose was born healthy, and soon became so plump and rosy that my meat-eating friends began to marvel at her health rather than worry about it!

"Tara is now two months old. I have entirely cut dairy out of my diet since, when I did eat it, Tara would break out in little red dots all over her chest. I have received zero comments about my diet since her birth, and our Naturopath is supportive and educated about vegetarianism. I look forward to raising our children on a vegetarian diet."

Valerie and Randy; babies Morgan, Zoe, Raven, and Mariah (California)

In 1989, Randy became vegan, Valerie became lacto-vegetarian, and their first two children became lacto-ovo vegetarian. Raven (born in 1988) and Mariah (born in 1991) have been weaned onto a lacto-ovo vegetarian diet. Valerie writes:

"Having a vegetarian baby was much easier than I expected. My earlier, meat-eating babies actually didn't like meat at first and had to be taught to eat it. I often disguised meat by mixing it into foods they liked, such as rice or potatoes. I since have learned that tofu is a marvelous baby food: bland, nutritious, squishy, adaptable, and non-staining. It's also nice not to have to worry during publicized outbreaks [of *E. coli*] from hamburgers (although we felt badly for the families who were harmed by bacteria).

"All babies should be nursed if at all possible!! We are certain this accounts for the excellent health (so far) of our four children. I tandem-nursed my last two children, and my vegetarian diet maintained a plentiful milk supply. My last baby—my only completely vegetarian pregnancy—was my smallest, but at 7 pounds, 15 ounces was completely healthy, and still is.

"A baby only knows what you feed him or her. For this reason, it's important for a vegetarian parent to spend as much time as possible with a baby. You know best and you love best for your child. Otherwise, you can spend a lot of time regretting the ignorance of your wishes on the part of caregivers. For example, my dad, for the life of him, couldn't accept that I didn't feed my children jello. Grandparents also worry a lot about babies not eating puréed meats out of jars. The only thing that reassures them is the good health and development of their grandchildren, not research or statistics."

Marcia; babies Tahira and Karaena (Washington)
Marcia has been a vegetarian since 1968. She experimented with a raw foods diet in the 1970s and has been vegan since 1976. Her daughters were born in 1984 and 1987, and have been raised as vegans. Tahira was one of the children featured in Dr. Klaper's book, *Pregnancy, Children, and the Vegan Diet*. Marcia writes:

"Both babies were 'off the charts!' The joke was that they were at the 200th percentile. Tahira had Loma Linda soymilk in addition to breast milk. The second time around, I had more knowledge and support for nursing, and Karaena only had mother's milk. She nursed until she was four years and four months.

"I never made 'baby food.' When they could eat a banana or avocado or a naturally soft food, I gave it to them. I never spoon-fed anything, nor did I feed them grains until they broke their first molars.

"Tahira was very strong for her age, spoke in full sentences at 16 and a half months, and at age two had the vocabulary of a five-year-old. She never 'toddled' and was very tall for her age until around age 12. Now she's 5'7" which seems to be average to 'average-tall' for her peer group of 14-year-olds. Karaena is so strong that her ballet teacher can't believe her musculature."

Jill and Steve; babies Adam and Leah (Georgia)

Jill and Steve have been vegetarians since 1983. Adam was born in 1993 and Leah in 1996, and both are being raised on a "mostly vegan" diet. Jill writes:

"I feel very strongly that raising my children as vegetarians helps them in two major ways. First, from birth their bodies are nourished by foods that come from positive, healthy sources— foods you can call by their real names because you don't have to hide where they come from. Second, their souls are nourished by the knowledge that it's not necessary to kill animals to survive.

"Two sets of obstetricians and pediatricians have been supportive of our lifestyle. The fact that both of our children are robust and healthy dispels a lot of pre-conceived notions. Neither has had the ear infections so common in our friends' children, and they rarely need to see a doctor aside from regular checkups.

"We felt very fortunate to have commercial vegetarian baby foods available. The hardest thing now that they're older is restaurant food; toddlers and young children can be picky eaters, and when the menu is already very limited for meatless options, sometimes you just have to let them get by on French fries and fruit until you get home. School lunches are largely a nightmare, just overloaded with meat and cheese. It's no wonder so many kids are overweight and unhealthy.

"The Vegetarian Society of Georgia recently started a monthly playgroup so that the kids can get together and be around children whose lifestyles match their own. I hope that subtle things like that now will help them deal with whatever overt peer pressure they might encounter when they're older.

"Adam may be the only vegetarian in his kindergarten class, but he never questions his diet, only other people's. He says, 'Mommy, if we just take vegetarian hamburgers to the grocery store, then everybody will see them and not buy the ones made out of dead cows.' And the other day when he was playing with his toy dinosaurs and toy people, he told me that the dinosaurs didn't eat the vegetarian people because they knew the vegetarians wouldn't hurt the other animals. The meat-eating people, however, were dinosaur lunch!"

Gena and Kevin; babies Geneva and K.J. (Georgia)

Gena has been vegan for 21 years, and Kevin for eight years. Their children, born in 1994 and 1998, are being raised as vegans. Gena writes:

"My children have been vegetarian from birth. Both breast-fed: my daughter till [she was] two and three-quarter years and who knows how long for my son. Neither has ever had cows' milk.

"My daughter is taller and weighs more than other non-vegetarian friends of the same age. She is soon to be four years old, and is already doing kindergarten and first-grade work on her computer at home. My son has never been on the 'growth charts' at the doctor's office. At eight months, he is the size of a one-and-a-half-year-old, and extremely healthy. And they say that vegetarian kids are smaller! Both kids are in great physical shape and have never been seriously ill.

"My daughter has no problem eating what we eat. She loves all the typical vegetarian food like hummus, tofu, raw vegetables, soy milk, nuts, grains, etc. She understands why she is vegetarian and tries to educate others about it. I am very proud of my food choices for my children."

Lynn and David; baby Flint (Washington)

Lynn has been lacto-ovo vegetarian since 1976, and David since 1982. Flint was born in 1988 and was weaned onto a lacto-ovo diet. Lynn writes:

"My son was born by C-section when I was 38 years old. He was 22" long and 8.5 pounds, and his weight/height has been off the charts ever since. I breast-fed Flint for over two and a half years, and by that age, most people mistook him for at least four. He has never tasted red meat, fish, or poultry, and eats an egg or two a week (from a friend's free-roaming chickens) along with occasional dairy products. By age eight, my son's foot could no longer squeeze into my shoes! And now, at age ten, he is 5'2" and weighs 115 pounds.

"From ages two to four, Flint was a very picky eater, rejecting many of the foods my husband and I liked best. These days I pack his lunch for school and include a salad with a separate bottle of oil and vinegar, vegetarian chili, crackers, and apple or pear, and a cocoa soy drink. For dinner, he can easily eat as much as an adult, and he loves salad and is a fan of spicy foods like curries, Mexican dishes, and cloves of garlic.

"If families create a solid base of values at home, peer pressure will have a minimal effect on their vegetarian children. Flint attends an alternative school, so there are other vegetarian kids there, and a couple of his friends are trying out a veggie diet based on his enthusiasm. His school lunches, while a little more labor-intensive, are the envy of kids and adults alike. He has never met anyone who has put down or made fun of his diet. And when my husband and I recently talked half-seriously about introducing seafood back into our diets, our son was outraged, saying he'd never eat the stuff. We're proud of him."

Jana and Michael; babies Crosby and Glacier (Alaska)
Jana became a vegetarian in 1989 and a vegan one year later. Her husband eats the plant-based diet she prepares with the addition of some wild game he hunts himself. Their children, born in 1991 and 1994, are being raised as vegans. Jana writes:

"Being a vegan in Alaska hasn't always been an easy adventure, especially when raising vegan children. The hard part is that we know no other vegan children or adults. I'm on my own quest in raising my vegan children. When birthdays or parties happen, I make the food for the situation. It's important to me that my children never feel left out.

"My pregnancies were very easy, and I worked hard in the way of building my babies from conception. With Crosby, I did a protein drink each morning, grinding sesame seeds and almonds to add to my soymilk, frozen banana, and protein powder. At one point my midwives (both boys were successfully born in our cabin) wanted me to take desiccated liver pills for iron, but I said, 'No thanks, I'll up my iron foods!' I did, and was very successful at bringing up my iron count.

"Crosby has always been over 100 percent on the growth chart for height and weight. His mind works beautifully as does his body. He is an amazing child, and I'm not just saying that because he is my son.

"Glacier was born after one and a half hours of labor, and he too was healthy and strong, which meant even more because he has Down's Syndrome. He did not have to be transported anywhere, and he nursed soon after being born! He continued to nurse until three and a half years. Both my boys were big nursers. Neither had a bottle although I tried with pumped milk, but I believe they wouldn't take that artificial nipple—they wanted the real thing!

"Glacier is an incredible Down's person, and others who deal with special needs children say that, too. His health is great, and he has never had an ear infection, which Down's babies are prone to, nor many colds.

"When people (including my husband, who goes along with the ride, but really isn't into it), say, 'Eating that just one time won't hurt them,' I say, 'One time probably won't hurt them, but I don't want them eating it; if you let them one time, how can they decide yes and no, now and then. It's too confusing.'"

Cindy and Rick; baby Vienna (Washington)

Cindy and Rick began eating a vegan diet in January of 1991. Vienna was born in the summer of 1998 and will be weaned to a vegan diet. Cindy writes:

"Initially, we started eating a vegetarian diet for health reasons. I love to cook, and for me it has been a wonderful adventure to learn how to prepare plant-based foods. Now, we continue to eat a vegan diet, not only for our own health, but also the health of the planet and out of compassion for animals. As the parents of a four-month-old baby girl, it is even more vitally important to us. We shop almost exclusively at the local co-op, and belong to an organic Community Supported Agriculture (CSA) farm.

"By the time I was pregnant, we had already been eating a vegan diet for almost seven years. We became active members of EarthSave, and so we have had lots of exposure to other parents who are raising their children vegetarian. In our EarthSave circle of friends, there is no skepticism at all. Our family's primary care physician is a Naturopathic doctor who raises his own children on a vegetarian diet! Even our parents, both sets, are okay with our choice. Probably the most common concern is, if we and the baby will be getting enough protein and calcium. When we explain that we get plenty of both from nuts, greens, tofu, avocado, grains, etc., the conversation ends.

"When I became pregnant, I did become more conscientious about eating plenty of protein-rich plant foods. I also took a vegan pre-natal supplement. I passed every single blood test that was required, and my neighbors were amazed at how active I was up until the birth. After Vienna's birth, I recovered quickly and lost the weight easily. I'm sure that breast-feeding helped with that.

"Vienna has been breast-fed from day one. She started out at seven pounds seven ounces and doubled that by three months. She has been in the 95th percentile for weight since the second-month checkup. Not a day goes by that someone does not comment about how healthy and happy she looks. At birth, she lifted her head up and nursed within the first 45 minutes. She was able to hold her head up on her own from about the sixth week, and is alert and well-organized."

Bonnie and Arthur; babies Jacob and Ryan (Virginia)
Bonnie and Arthur have been vegan since 1995. Their children,

born in 1994 and 1998, are being raised as vegans. Bonnie writes:

"In college, I experimented with vegetarian days. Then, while living with my future husband, I started an every-other-day vegetarian diet.

"When I became pregnant with my first child, I began reading books about nursing, and decided breast-feeding was absolutely the only way I would feed my child. Both my husband and I were very allergic as children—[my allergies] taking the form of asthma and bronchitis and my husband's as skin problems. We were both allergic to cows' milk as infants, and our mothers had difficulty finding formulas to agree with us. My husband was having terrible breakouts of eczema, and sometimes would have three or four fingers with band-aids on them, so he decided to cut dairy products out of his diet, and his eczema disappeared. But I was frantic to get enough calcium and so was adding non-fat dry milk to my milk at night and eating four Tums every night as well (as per the doctor).

"Jacob was born in September, and nursing was great. I had decided to nurse exclusively for six months since I had read that early introduction of solids was implicated in food allergies. At six months, he received a DT inoculation and within two hours broke out in a rash. I decided not to introduce solids until he was nine months old.

"Then, in May, our family went to a La Leche League conference where the keynote speaker was Jay Gordon, M.D. After hearing him speak, and reading his book, we were convinced we wanted to raise our son as a vegan. Jacob then decided for himself, at eight and a half months, to help himself to a roll from the bread basket, so we started him with sweet potatoes and other vegetables and fruits. Then grains.

"When I became pregnant again, I found a vegetarian dietitian who reviewed two weeks of food diaries and said she had never seen such a well-rounded diet. I grew a beautiful, healthy, 8 pound 14 ounce baby. Ryan continues to be way off the charts for growth, and both my children are incredibly healthy. Our pediatrician wishes more women would nurse long-term."

Dianne and Lee; baby Mitchell (Colorado)

Dianne became a lacto-ovo vegetarian in 1974 while Lee eats a vegetarian diet "sometimes." Mitchell was born in 1989, and was weaned onto a lacto-ovo vegetarian diet. Dianne writes:

"Mitchell weighed 17 pounds by four months, and now, at almost ten years, he weighs close to 90 pounds—not fat, but solid and muscular. He rarely had ear infections—compared to other kids—and rarely misses school due to illness.

"When he was a baby, we bought organic baby foods. He never would accept a bottle except for juice. Mitchell has never found a vegetable he doesn't like, although he is not too fond of avocados. His favorite vegetables are eggplant and turnips, and he has always liked salads. For a while, his favorite food was plain cheese pizza—now he says it's lasagna.

"We never had any difficulty in raising a vegetarian child. The pediatrician was okay with it. The obstetrician had been vegetarian previously, and when my weight gain during pregnancy was good, he never had any problems with my diet. My parents were somewhat skeptical, but Mitchell is their only grandchild who is not a picky eater."

Susanne and Jim; babies Jordan and Evan (Washington)

Susanne has been vegetarian for "most of the time since childhood" and vegan since 1994. Jim became vegan in 1988. Their daughter was born in 1996 and was weaned onto a vegan diet. Their son was born in 1998 and is still nursing. Susanne writes:

"It is funny that people are concerned about the health of children on a vegan diet. All the people I know that have small children who are eating the Standard American Diet have kids who are always sick. My friends and I, with vegan kids, have kids who are very rarely sick. Jordan has never been sick except for mild colds. People should be worried about the non-vegan children."

Interview Statistics

As noted above, not all the respondents included personal stories, but all included at least some data concerning themselves and their children. The informal questionnaire that was sent elicited the following basic information:

Data were obtained for 40 children from 25 families in 12 states.

The ages of the children ranged from less than two months to nearly 16 years (as of November of 1998).

The average weight at birth for 35 of the children was 7 pounds 4 ounces, with a high of 10 pounds 4 ounces and a low of 6 pounds 4 ounces. (Compare that to the "healthy average" of between 5 pounds 11.5 ounces and 8 pounds 5.75 ounces.)[15]

The average length at birth for 32 of the children was 20.67 inches, with a high of 23 inches and a low of 19 inches.

The average Apgar score at birth for 18 of the children was 9, with a high of 10 and a low of 2 (for a child born with the umbilical cord around its neck). Only one birth was reported to be a Caesarean section, and one as premature. (The Apgar tests help the doctor assess the baby's condition at birth but do not predict later health or development. Most children born in the U.S. receive an Apgar score of between 8 and 10, but "few score a perfect 10."[16]

As reported by those parents answering the question, 29 of the children were exclusively breast-fed, and eight were both breast- and bottle-fed to varying degrees. None was reported to be exclusively bottle-fed.

The average age at introduction of solids for 32 children was 6.6 months, with a high of 12 months and a low of 5 weeks.

The average age at final weaning for 21 children was 29.4 months, with a high of 4.5 years and a low of 11 months.

The diet upon weaning was identified to be vegan for 12 children; "near-vegan" for three children; lacto-ovo vegetarian for ten children; macrobiotic for two children; pisco-pollarian for two children; and omnivorous for two children (they were not included in the above data analysis).

One lacto-ovo vegetarian child became vegan at 21 months. The two omnivorous children became vegetarian at five and seven years. Of the children not yet weaned, their parents expressed the intention of weaning them to a lacto-ovo vegetarian diet in one case, and a vegan diet in five others.

Twenty-six of the children were reported to be in "excellent" health; seven to be in "good" health; and one to be of "average" health. Two children were reported to suffer from allergies to dairy products. One child was reported to be allergic to nuts and to suffer from mild asthma. Finally, one pregnancy resulted in a miscarriage, and as noted in the interviews, one child has Down's Syndrome.

The conclusion? Vegetarians are "just plain folks" who lead lives that are as ordinary as possible given the constraints imposed by the surrounding non-vegetarian culture. And while vegetarianism certainly is not a panacea, these families amply demonstrate that it is possible to have children who develop normally—mentally, physically, and emotionally—on both lacto-ovo vegetarian and vegan diets. In other words, as was stated in the introduction to this book, not only can children be fed a vegetarian diet from birth, but they can *thrive* on it!

Table 3.1: RDA During Pregnancy and Lactation[17]

	ADULT WOMEN 25–50 YEARS	PREGNANT WOMEN 25–50 YEARS	LACTATING WOMEN 25–50 YEARS 0–6 MONTHS	LACTATING WOMEN 25–50 YEARS 6–12 MONTHS
Energy *(kcal)*	2200	+300	+500	+50
Protein *(g)*	50	60	65	62
Vitamin A *(micrograms RE)*	800	800	1300	1200
Vitamin E *(milligrams α-TE)*	8	10	12	11
Vitamin K *(micrograms)*	65	65	65	65
Vitamin C *(milligrams)*	60	70	95	90
Iron *(milligrams)*	15	30	15	15
Zinc *(milligrams)*	12	15	19	16
Iodine *(micrograms)*	15	17	20	20

Table 3.2: DRI During Pregnancy and Lactation[18]

	ADULT WOMEN 19–30 YEARS	ADULT WOMEN 31–50 YEARS	PREGNANT WOMEN 19–30 YEARS	PREGNANT WOMEN 31–50 YEARS	LACTATING WOMEN 19–30 YEARS	LACTATING WOMEN 31–50 YEARS
Vitamin D (micrograms)	5	5	5	5	5	5
Calcium (milligrams)	1000	1000	1000	1000	1000	1000
Phosphorus (milligrams)	700	700	700	700	700	700
Magnesium (milligrams)	310	320	350	360	310	320
Fluoride (milligrams)	3	3	3	3	3	3
Thiamin (milligrams)	1.1	1.1	1.4	1.4	1.5	1.5
Riboflavin (milligrams)	1.1	1.1	1.4	1.4	1.6	1.6
Niacin (milligrams NE)	14	14	18	18	17	17
Vitamin B-6 (milligrams)	1.3	1.5	2.0	1.9	2.2	2.0
Biotin (micrograms)	30	30	30	30	35	35
Choline (milligrams)	425	425	450	450	550	550
Pantothenic Acid (milligrams)	5	5	6	6	7	7
Folate (micrograms)	400	400	600	600	500	500
Vitamin B-12 (micrograms)	2.4	2.4	2.6	2.6	2.8	2.8

Food Guide for Pregnant and Lactating Vegetarians

Strive to eat the number of servings listed for each group daily, choosing a variety of foods from within each group. The number of servings may be increased if necessary for adequate (but not excessive) weight gain during pregnancy and to maintain energy and milk supply during lactation. Consider taking a vegetarian vitamin/mineral supplement formulated for pregnancy and lactation to ensure full nutrition, especially if your appetite is poor. This servings guide is adapted from the following sources:

The guide in the original *Vegetarian Baby,* which was in turn adapted from the *Birth and Family Journal* (v3, p. 85) and *Laurel's Kitchen* by Laurel Robertson (*out of print*).

Food Guides for Pregnant and Breast-feeding Vegetarians in *The Dietitian's Guide to Vegetarian Diets: Issues and Applications* by Mark Messina Ph.D. and Virginia Messina, MPH, RD, p. 256.

Pregnancy, Children, and the Vegan Diet by Michael Klaper, MD.

Food Guides for the Vegetarian, by P.B. Mutch, in the *American Journal of Clinical Nutrition* 1998; 48:913-919.

Please remember that this is just a guide—not the law! If your body demands you eat differently from what is outlined here, listen to your instincts. And if you have any questions, please discuss them with your doctor or a nutritionist.

Lacto-Ovo Vegetarian Servings Guide

	LEGUMES	GRAINS	VEGETABLES	FRUITS	NUTS AND SEEDS	DAIRY PRODUCTS AND EGGS†
Pregnant	2	6	4	4	1	4
Lactating	3	7	5	4	1	4

† *Maximum of four eggs per week*

Vegan Servings Guide
(include a reliable vitamin B-12 source)

	LEGUMES	GRAINS	VEGETABLES	FRUITS	NUTS AND SEEDS	SOY PRODUCTS*
Pregnant	2	6	4	4	1	4
Lactating	3	7	5	4	1	4

* *Soy milk and soy-based meat analogues, preferably fortified. If you are allergic to soy, increase the servings in all of the other groups except fruits.*

Standard Servings Sizes for Adults

Legumes
   beans, dried peas, lentils (1/2 cup, cooked)
   tofu, tempeh (4 ounces)
   soy milk (1 cup)
   soy yogurt (1 cup)

Grains
   whole grains (1/2 cup, cooked)
   pasta (1/2 cup, cooked)
   cold cereal (1 ounce)
   bread (1 slice)

Vegetables
   dark green leafy (1/2 cup, cooked)
   leafy salad (1 cup, raw)
   chopped (1/2 cup, raw)
   sea vegetables (1 ounce, dried)
   juice (4 ounces)

Fruits
   whole (1 medium-sized)
   cooked (1/2 cup)
   juice (4 ounces)
   dried (1 ounce)

Nuts and Seeds
   whole nuts (1 ounce)
   whole seeds (2 tablespoons)
   nut and seed butters (2 tablespoons)

Dairy Products
   cows' or goats' milk (1 cup)
   cows' milk yogurt (1 cup)
   hard cheese (1 ounce)
   cottage cheese (1 cup)

Eggs (1 medium)

Development and Diet

SHARON'S STORY: *Academic Curiosity*

My academic background is in child development, so naturally I am very interested in the relationship between the social and physiological aspects of eating. I also wanted to know answers to questions such as "When can you feed a baby tofu?" and "Why is a baby ready for beans at around ten months of age, but not before?" The early maturing process, both physical and social, is complex and exciting. It is a time to relax and enjoy the changes rather than a time to try to rush a child to the next stage.

• • •

THE RELATIONSHIP between internal development and eating habits usually is not described in most baby books, but an understanding of this connection can help parents to see such things as why some foods are best eaten after eight months, or even 12 months of age, or why breast-feeding should take place on a demand schedule rather than on a fixed schedule. The natural timing between the development of a baby's various physical abilities and the growing expectations for appropriate social behavior is truly amazing—although perhaps it really should not be so surprising when viewed in the light of thousands of generations of trial and error on the part of parents!

As an example, the development of good hand-to-mouth control coincides with the time when a baby is expected to begin self-feeding, and it is at this same time that a baby begins to display a strong desire to feed himself or herself. Observing such links between behavior and development can be a special delight for all parents.

Before Birth

Prenatally, infants have the ability to suck; infants can be seen by ultrasound sucking their thumbs . . . [and] by 37 weeks, the combination of sucking, swallowing, and breathing is well coordinated.[1]

Somewhere between the third and the fifth months of pregnancy, the digestive system of the fetus is developed well enough for the fetus to begin swallowing amniotic fluid and for the intestines to begin absorbing a small amount of protein from that source.[2] The taste buds also are developed well enough by four and a half months for the fetus to begin to distinguish between the "different tastes . . . [of] amniotic fluid, which includes glucose, lactic acid, and urea."[3] At the same time, peristalsis begins in the small intestine, followed by development of the sucking reflex at around six months of gestation. Premature infants often have not developed this reflex fully at the time of birth which can make it more difficult for them to nurse for the first few days or weeks of life.[4]

Birth to One Month

The colostrum from the breast primes the digestive tract, emptying the meconium and leaving a coating of immunizing properties.[5]

The first item on any baby's menu is colostrum, closely followed by milk. Most babies need nothing more for several months because their digestive systems are designed specifically for this food.

The newborn has four reflexes that help bring milk into the body. The first—the rooting reflex—causes a baby to turn its head and to reach with the lips toward any pressure applied to the cheeks. The smell of milk also can help direct a baby's lips when the breast is near. The tongue extrusion and sucking reflexes help the baby latch onto the nipple and pull milk into the back of the mouth. The swallowing reflex then passes the milk into the esophagus, where muscular contractions push it into the stomach.[6]

Digestion begins when the milk mixes with the saliva, which contains alpha-amylase, a starch-splitting enzyme. Infants have lower concentrations of amylase in both saliva and pancreas than adults, however, and there is little time for the newborn's saliva to begin to digest food because the swallowing reflex quickly pushes the food down into the stomach. Nature, therefore, has designed breast milk to include amylase so digestion of starch and glucose can proceed efficiently. This amylase survives the low acid levels in the infant stomach and continues the process of digestion in the intestinal tract.[7]

In the stomach, high pH levels, low production of pepsin, and protease inhibitors in colostrum and milk, inhibit protein digestion in newborns, but this gradually changes as pH levels start to fall between two to six weeks.[8] The casein in human milk also has "chemical properties . . . [that] promote the formation of a soft, flocculent curd, which is easier for human infants to digest than the casein in other animals' milk."[9] Fats are more easily digested than protein as lipase enzymes are present in colostrum and breast milk and are produced by the tongue, the stomach, the pancreas, and the duodenum. The pancreatic lipase is relatively low in newborns, but it increases rapidly during the first month. Bile acids also are low to start with, but they are present in enough quantity to activate the lipase in breast milk to the point where 90 to 95 percent of the fat is absorbed.[10-11]

Within five to ten minutes after food enters a newborn's stomach, it starts to empty into the duodenum, the first part of the small intestine. Half of the milk will have left the stomach within approximately thirty to seventy minutes with the stomach being completely emptied within two to three hours.[12] Infants, therefore, will want to nurse every two to three hours during the first few weeks which is why rigid feeding schedules should be avoided.

Meanwhile, in the duodenum, pancreatic juices and bile continue to digest the milk while trypsin acts on the partially digested proteins, breaking them into their component amino acids which then can be used by the body. Trypsin levels are low at birth, but gradually increase to "the levels of older children" by six months.[13]

The primary carbohydrate in milk, lactose, is digested by an intestinal enzyme called lactase. The amount of lactase in the digestive juices increases before birth and reaches its highest level during the early weeks of life, decreasing considerably after weaning, with the timing and amount of decrease largely depending on ethnicity.[14] At no other time during life can lactose be as easily and efficiently digested as during the nursing period.

To complete the digestive process, other less prevalent carbohydrates are digested by enzymes present in the duodenum such as sucrase, maltase, and gluco-amylase, which reach mature levels somewhere between birth and the end of the first month.[15-16] Leftover lactose also can become available after fermentation by colon bacteria, but more complex carbohydrates such as starch are not as well digested during the first six months of life as they will be later.[17] In contrast, vitamin B-12, and some minerals such as iron and zinc, are absorbed more efficiently in babies than adults.[18-19]

After the nutrients are absorbed during their passage through the intestine, the indigestible food residues are deposited in the lower end of the gastrointestinal tract for excretion—a fact with which parents become all too familiar within a short time after birth!

To increase the efficiency of digestion, a mother's milk supply varies in response to her baby's needs, which change from day to day. A newborn's stomach can hold only about an ounce of fluid, but within ten days the stomach's capacity increases to almost three and one-half ounces. By one month of age, the baby's stomach can hold six ounces at one time. Likewise, a mother has almost no milk in her breasts when the baby is born, but her supply increases dramatically over the first few weeks. In addition, the composition of the mother's milk changes as the baby becomes better able to digest fats and carbohydrates. As you can see, mother's milk is the ideal diet for the baby.

In addition to providing optimal nutrition, breast-feeding also helps the baby to develop a healthy digestive tract which in turn results in a strong immune system. The mucous lining of the digestive tract shields the body from foreign proteins and pathogens, but an infant's intestines are relatively permeable and need time to form such a barrier. Until the mucous lining is completely developed, a child will be very vulnerable to allergens and food-poisoning organisms. Increased acidity in the stomach and other factors also must develop before the infant is safely able to digest foods other than breast milk. In addition, breast milk helps colonize the infant's digestive tract with beneficial intestinal flora such as bifido-bacteria, and transfers immunity through immunoglobulins and other defense factors.[20-21] Finally, breast milk contains a diverse array of hormones.[22]

Obviously no formula will offer all the benefits of breast milk, but formulas can be a satisfactory substitute for mother's milk when an alternative is necessary. However, a few special considerations must be taken when bottle-feeding instead of breast-feeding a baby. Nursing from a bottle requires more control of the swallowing reflex than does nursing at the breast, since the breast's letdown reflex assists the baby by spurting out milk at intervals. This spurting is somewhat controlled by the baby's way of nursing. Small, quick movements bring more milk, and gulping slows down the flow. If you watch your baby closely, you will notice that he or she alternates these movements. When the breast spurts milk, the swallowing reflex works most efficiently and the baby takes in little air. A bottle is not so responsive. As a result, bottle-fed babies will need more burping than breast-fed babies.

Another consideration for the bottle-fed baby relates to milk intake over time. A baby will empty a breast quickly, and spend the majority of time at the breast sucking and strengthening the jaws and mouth. A bottle-fed baby continues to get food as long as he or she sucks and may swallow more food than is necessary in order to satisfy important sucking needs. If your baby is bottle-fed, you may need to regulate the amount of milk your baby drinks in order to avoid overfeeding. The six to eight ounces that a one-month-old baby usually takes at a feeding can be given in a bottle with a "preemie" nipple, which will reduce the amount of milk that can be sucked at one time. This will extend the time for sucking without increasing the amount the baby is fed.

Contrary to popular belief, taste is not a factor in the choice between breast milk and formula. As noted above, taste buds are present at birth, and a baby can discriminate tastes at that time, but mature connections between the taste buds and the brain do not become established for several months. Babies do show a decided preference for sweet, however, and according to one study, "This preference continues as long as sweetened [sugar] solution is offered, and preference at age two is significantly correlated to the amount of solution consumed at six months of age. If sweetened water is not offered after birth, there seems to be a diminished acceptability to it."[23]

Although breast-feeding certainly is optimal in most cases, don't be discouraged if you cannot breast-feed because of health concerns, adoption, or some other reason. As described above, bottle feeding requires a little more thought than breast-feeding, but it will provide the nourishment your baby needs if a quality formula is used. In either case, if you are relaxed and loving while you feed your baby, you are creating the beginning of a good attitude towards food and eating.

One to Four Months

As a baby grows, his or her feeding habits change. The stomach is growing, so the baby drinks more milk. The quantity and quality of mother's milk changes to accommodate the baby's needs. The fat content of the milk increases, slowing digestion and thereby increasing the amount of time between feedings. More complex carbohydrates appear in quantity, and the baby's digestive system matures, producing more of the starch-splitting enzymes.

Because digestion is slowing down, and because food remains in the stomach longer, your baby's feeding requests will probably occur less frequently, often at intervals of three hours or more. He or she might nurse longer in the evening, in preparation for a longer sleeping period at night. Your baby naturally develops a feeding schedule suited to his or her needs, eventually approaching adult patterns as the months proceed. Again, rigid routines are not necessary.

In addition to developments that immediately affect feeding, babies grow in ways that will later contribute to changes in diet. They begin to hold their heads erect, they can control their eyes, and they begin to swipe at objects, making contact with them by the end of this period.

Four to Six Months

Beginning at four months and no later than six months, the infant is gradually introduced to weaning foods. The order of introduction is not precise and schedules will vary since each infant will progress at his/her own rate.[24]

By the time a baby is four months old, his or her vision has matured. Your baby now anticipates food when a breast or bottle comes into view. Because depth perception is enhanced, eye-hand coordination improves greatly. For example, your baby can see you holding a bottle, reach for it, hold it, and possibly maneuver it into his or her mouth. No longer does your baby respond only to breast or bottle closeness; vision has become more important than the oral reflex in exciting appetite.

During this time, you may notice that your baby nurses for shorter periods of time than before—a behavior some people call "suck and run." Your baby sees new things to explore, and his or her attention doesn't stay focused on eating. Because the breast is responsive to the length of sucking time, the milk supply decreases, a change which heralds the need to supplement your baby's diet with other foods. This is a special time for your partner, who now can become fully involved in feeding the baby as weaning begins.

Although the baby can begin to eat foods, only a few specially prepared solids are appropriate. The baby still has poor control over the swallowing reflex, and when fed solids, pushes the tongue out and closes the lips at the "wrong" time, appearing to spit out the food. These actions are not a rejection of the taste of the food, but rather the results of immature coordination, which practice—in the short run—improves only slightly. One guideline used by many parents is only to offer foods that are easily mashed by hand, such as soft, ripe fruits, while avoiding those where preparation involves the use of blenders and grinders (whether at home or during commercial baby food manufacture). You also can delay the introduction of solids until the sixth month.

Six to Nine Months

By the age of six months, a baby can eat solid foods, and delaying their introduction any longer can result in malnutrition and attendant problems.[25] Swallowing becomes voluntary; a baby can hold food in the mouth, spit it out, or swallow it at will. Pancreatic fluid and other digestive juices are nearly like an adult's and are able to digest more complex proteins and carbohydrates. The baby's ability to sit unaided has freed the hands to begin their exploratory development. The hands, as a result, become more flexible and versatile. The eyes and hands are well coordinated, allowing the child to grab at the food he or she is offered. Grabbing is the signal in many cultures to introduce solid foods to a child.

New foods should be added to the diet one at a time, with a few days between each, so that any allergic reactions or food sensitivities can be identified. By nine months of age, your baby will be able to digest most legumes, grains, fruits, and vegetables, if you soften or grind them first. Some foods should be avoided for the first year, however, either because they can contain botulism spores, their proteins are the ones most likely to create allergies, or they present a choking hazard. Details are given in the following chapters.

A baby food grinder, blender, or similar machine can produce soft, spoon-able food, even from raw vegetables and fruits. Christine Ripault, in *Children's Gastronomique,* suggests that you don't feed the more lumpy foods by spoon, but rather allow your child to pick them up with his or her fingers: " . . . if there should be a lump in the spoon-fed food, he is confused. He is accustomed to pushing spoon-fed food back to his throat and slipping it down. Lumps do not go this way, so not knowing how to manage a lump, the baby spits it out. However, if this same baby picks up an object in his fingers and puts it in his mouth, he will immediately begin to chew on it."[26]

It is during the period from six to nine months of age that a baby's teeth usually begin to appear. Your baby will probably want to chew on everything and to gnaw, actions which soothe irritated gums and help push the teeth through them to the surface. This is the time to offer "finger foods," such as pieces of fruit or biscuits, that your child can pick up and chew. Please note that finger foods are primarily for practice; they will not form a large part of the nutritional intake at this point. Make sure that finger foods are not too hard, large, sharp, or round to prevent swallowing problems. It is advisable to take a class on CPR for children so you will know what to do if your child swallows something wrong.

Finally, as a baby's taste buds and nervous system mature, likes and dislikes become apparent. After introducing foods one at a time to check for allergies, you should offer a variety of foods regularly on the premise that the wider your child's experience, the more easily new tastes and consistencies will be accepted. Rotating foods from different botanical groups also can help prevent the later development of allergies and food sensitivities.

It often will take three or four meals for your child to get used to a new taste, so don't be discouraged immediately if a food is rejected the first time out. Above all, do not force any foods on your baby; you might make him or her reject these foods more vehemently or permanently.

SHARON'S STORY: *Then and Now*

A rigid schedule for feeding babies was more common a generation ago than it is now. I found a schedule, reproduced here, that my parents' doctor gave them when I was nine months old. It outlines a very structured feeding practice and shows that I was eating complete meals by this age. This rigid structure is now known to be unnecessary, especially if a baby is still breast-fed. Breast-feeding is more common now than it was when I was young, which may contribute to such a full daily meal plan at so early an age. The pediatrician told my mother to stop breast-feeding me after three months.

As I look at this rigid schedule, so different from the way I feed my son, I realize that my parents must have given me an extra lot of love to balance such a constricting eating pattern. It makes me feel that the attitudes with which parents feed children are at least as important as the style of preparation.

.   .   .

Feeding Schedule at Nine Months of Age, 1952

Name _____ Age _____ Weight _____ Height _____

BREAKFAST, 7 TO 8 A.M.

1. Fruit Sauce—Apple, Prune, or Apricot; well-cooked and crushed through a sieve, one to three tablespoonfuls. Or juice of whole large orange or, after 18 months, juice of half grapefruit.
2. Cereal (cooked) three to six tablespoons. Pablum Mixed Cereal or Pablum Oatmeal (these require no cooking). Cream of wheat, oatmeal.
3. Toast or Bread (day-old) with Butter.
4. Hard- or Soft-Boiled or Coddled Egg yolk three times a week. Broiled Bacon occasionally.
5. Milk, eight to ten ounces from cup.

DINNER 12 TO 2 P.M.

1. Broth (clear) or thickened with rice or barley, or included in purée of Pea or Potato. Or creamed soups, or 8-10 ounces of whole milk.
2. Vegetable—Spinach, Carrots, Yellow Turnips, Beets, Peas, String or Wax Beans, Squash, Celery, or root Artichokes. After the second year, Cauliflower, Asparagus or Tomato (raw or stewed).
3. Potato (baked) or Spaghetti, Macaroni, Rice, or Hominy.
4. Bacon (broiled) after the _____ month. Calves Liver or Breast of Chicken after the _____ month. Lamb Chop or Beef (roast or steak) after the _____ month. Fish after the second year. All should be broiled or roasted—never fried.
5. Junket, Blanc Mange, Jello, Rice or Tapioca Pudding or Baked Apple. After eighteen months, Custard or Prune Whip or baked Banana. Occasionally Ice Cream.

SUPPER 5 TO 6 P.M.

1. Fruit Sauce (as given above). After second year, canned fruit.
2. Cereal, Rice, or Cornmeal Mush, three to six tablespoons.
3. Toast or Bread (day-old) with Butter, Honey, or Jelly.
4. Vegetables after second year.
5. Milk, eight to ten ounces from cup.

No Egg White or Anything Containing Egg White Before 18 Months of Age.

_____ Cod Liver Oil or _____ drops of

_____ _____ times daily.

Nine to Twelve Months

During this time, a child begins to move alone, to sit and stand steadily, and to develop better control of the hands. There is less sloppiness during eating because the child is able to put food into its mouth more accurately, preferring to pick things up with the forefinger and thumb rather than with an open-and-shut palming grasp. Children often go through a period of loving peas, firm tofu chunks, or similar foods because they can pick them up so neatly with their fingers and thumb, and put them cleanly into their mouths. Such control is satisfying—for the child and the parents.

There is more imitation during these months. Now that your baby has better body control, he or she can begin to watch others more closely and imitate their behavior. This is the right time to let your child experiment with a cup and spoon while you eat. Your child's interest and imitative ability allow social customs, like language, to be learned easily. Table etiquette begins at this age, but keep in mind that eating with the hands is important for babies, even through the second year of life. Allowing your child to use a spoon and a cup does not mean that he or she is ready physically or emotionally to master these skills. Above all, mealtime should be enjoyable, not rushed or overly disciplined. This is the time to enjoy your baby's development as an individual.

Variety continues to be important, not just for nutritional reasons, but because texture, color, and even attractiveness are becoming factors in your child's interest in food, as he or she grows aware of the finer details in the surrounding world.

Twelve to Twenty-four Months

During the second year of life, a baby learns to walk and talk as well as refining other motor and social skills. These new abilities coincide with the growth of a sense of independence and a desire to do things alone. The child wants to explore the things of the world more thoroughly than before and begins to distinguish social context. The highchair and the kitchen are places where the baby can exercise the combined growth of independence and motor skills.

When your child can talk and use his or her hands well, you will have a very eager assistant when preparing a meal. Filling measuring cups, pouring foods from one container to another, washing vegetables and fruits: all of these tasks will develop motor skills and give the child a sense of true importance. Helping with meal preparation teaches your child respect and love for food and creates a closeness with you because you share that process.

This also can be a good time to begin a child's garden with foods that are easy to plant and grow like garlic, sunflowers, radishes, squashes, lettuces, and runner beans. Children especially enjoy growing sprouts on a window sill. For an older child, trips to "U-pick" or Community Supported Agriculture (CSA) farms can further illustrate the connection between agriculture and food.

Constructive play with food can continue at the table. Although your child knows how to use a spoon and a fork, he or she still will want to explore shapes and textures with fingers. There is pleasure in pushing food into a spoon with the fingers before the food disappears into the mouth. There also is pleasure in using plant foods in playful artworks, such as stringing tube pasta into a necklace or making funny faces with vegetables as illustrated in the book, *Play With Your Food* by Joost Elffers (Stewart, Tabori, & Chang, 1997). Foods such as radishes and carrots can be nibbled on during such play and others cooked afterwards. Your child might even learn to like new foods after being introduced to them in this entertaining fashion.

Finally, even cleaning up after a meal can be a fun-filled learning experience if it is approached with an attitude of enjoyment by the entire family. Your child will be proud to help you by being given the responsibility of wiping the table with a cloth and dunking bowls and cups into warm, sudsy water in the sink.

Once your child learns to talk, a new level of communication opens. Your child can tell you about liking and hating foods.

Because imitation is such a strong learning motivation at this time, you may hear your child voicing your own likes and dislikes, ones that you might have been trying to hide. I suspect that this period is often the start of the "My child hates vegetables" attitude. Out of a sense of duty, parents may try to feed a child vegetables they themselves heartily dislike. The child will usually learn to dislike those same vegetables quickly. Vegetarians will probably have much less trouble with this stage than do parents who have limited vegetable preferences. It has been found that most children do like vegetables, and during the second year much prefer raw vegetables to cooked ones. Vegetarians who enjoy a wide variety of vegetables probably will discover this vegetable "trick" quickly.

Interest in food actually can be created by conversation with the one- to two-year-old child. Comparing colors, talking about where the food comes from, and discussing preparation for a meal may help a child try a new food that might otherwise be passed up for a familiar one. In general, helping a child to enjoy a meal and to respect the food which is eaten will assure good eating habits and health.

As your child observes and imitates you more closely, he or she will prefer to eat what you eat rather than a separately prepared meal. You will find this an excellent opportunity to gradually switch him or her to an adult menu, but remember that your child may not yet have the teeth necessary to chew all foods.

Evaluating Growth Rates

Fels data from birth to age 3 years [used for growth charts since 1977] were derived mainly from formula-fed infants . . . . Replacing the Fels data for infants with national survey data collected from 1971 to 1994 will better represent the combined growth patterns of breast-fed and formula-fed infants.[27]

The lower preadolescent height reported here, the possible delayed onset of the growth spurt, and the later age of menarche observed in lacto-ovo vegetarian girls all indicate a chronological delay in physical maturation. This maturation delay may carry potential health benefits in adult life. A later age of menarche has been consistently associated with decreased risk for several cancers, particularly of the breast.[28]

As was discussed in the first chapter, babies who are fed inadequate diets can experience retarded growth and failure to thrive due to malnutrition. This problem certainly is not limited to vegetarians; the majority of the world's people is omnivorous, so malnutrition obviously is not magically cured by animal foods. But because of our own society's fear of vegetarian diets, much publicity has focused on those vegetarians who have, through ignorance, fed their babies poorly, sometimes with disastrous results.

In evaluating information about children's development, one has to ask what constitutes a "normal" growth rate. Growth charts are themselves derived from data taken from growing children. As an example, in the United Kingdom, "Data from the 1990 survey of the National Study of Health and Growth, comprising 3,357 white English boys and 3,050 white English girls, were used to construct and evaluate a new index of weight-for-height."[29] Will children with different ethnic backgrounds "measure up" when evaluated according to such a chart? According to the National Center For Health Statistics (NCHS), they will: "Both current knowledge and expert opinion indicate that all children have a similar genetic potential for growth. Observed racial/ethnic differences in growth appear to be attributable primarily to environmental influences."[30] Because of this consensus, the charts developed in the United States "have been adapted by the World Health Organization for international use."[31]

Given that, it is a relief to know that children can and do grow normally on vegetarian diets that follow guidelines such as those presented in this book. Even so, the growth pattern of healthy vegetarian children might be slightly different from that of their omnivorous peers, and both parents and health care workers need to be aware of that possibility. For example, vegetarian children tend to be significantly thinner than omnivorous children. Given our all too rapidly "expanding" population, this can be perceived to be an advantage. Some studies also have found vegetarian children to be slightly shorter than average—something on the order of one inch.[32] These slightly lower average heights are still well within normal range, however, and "catch-up" growth may occur before or during adolescence. In fact, at least one study found older vegetarian children to be taller, on average, than their omnivorous counterparts.[33] Doctors and others would do well to remember that "[growth] charts are intended to serve as growth references, rather than as growth standards or clinical ideals to be achieved."[34]

Your child is likely to grow at a normal rate according to accepted charts if you offer a diet which includes plentiful protein and fat as well as being rich in vitamins and minerals. (*Note:* For the latest growth charts check the National Health and Nutrition Examination Survey website at http://www.cdc.gov/nchswww.)

The slightly smaller average stature of vegetarian children which may have been observed in the past might not be observed in the future as more vegetarians learn how best to feed their families. Many of the people interviewed for chapter three reported excellent growth rates for their children. One mother even proudly supplied her son's growth chart, which has been reproduced here. It gives an excellent example of how a vegan/vegetarian child can indeed grow, grow, grow!

Growth Chart for Jeffrey, Vegan Since 14 Months of Age

Born 1991; Apgar Score at birth: 9

Background: Breast-fed; first solids at 6 months; weaned to vegan diet at 14 months.

General health excellent. Has had colds, but never an ear infection or any serious illness. Mother and father both vegan since 1988.

AGE	WEIGHT / (PERCENTILE)	HEIGHT / (PERCENTILE)	HEAD CIRCUMFERENCE/ (PERCENTILE)*
0 month	7 pounds 12 ounces (50%)	20.50" (50%)	NA
1 month	8 pounds 12 ounces (75%)	21.25" (50%)	14.25"
2 months	12 pounds 4 ounces (75%)	23.25" (75%)	16.0"
4 months	15 pounds 5 ounces (50%)	24.75" (50%)	16.87"
6 months	19 pounds 3 ounces (75%)	26.75" (75%)	17.5" (60%)
9 months	22 pounds 11 ounces (75%)	29.0" (75%)	18.5" (80%)
12 months	24 pounds 3 ounces (75%)	30.0" (50%)	19.5" (90%)
15 months	26 pounds 11 ounces (75%)	31.5" (50%)	19.5" (90%)
18 months	27 pounds 15 ounces (75%)	33.25" (75%)	19.5" (90%)
24 months	31 pounds 4 ounces (75%)	35.0" (75%)	20.0" (90%)
4 years	40 pounds 5 ounces (75%)	40.5" (50%)	NA
5 years	44 pounds (50%)	42.75" (50%)	NA
6 years	47 pounds (75%)	44.5" (25%)	NA
7 years	52 pounds (75%)	48.0" (50%)	NA

* The percentiles given for head circumference are based on the values supplied by Jeffrey's parents from his medical records; those for weight and height have been confirmed or suitably amended according to the standard graphic charts reproduced in the *Pediatric Nutrition Handbook*, Fourth edition.

FIVE

Food Preparation

Eating should never be an obligation but rather one of the subtleties of good living.

Christine Ripault, *Children's Gastronomique*[1]

General Principles

SHARON'S STORY: *Finding the Right Foods*

Food selection and preparation is a vital and personal part of feeding a baby. I believe that knowing more about the foods you eat will make eating them more enjoyable. Respecting these natural gifts and the utensils that you use to prepare them is as important as any other aspect of feeding a baby. For example, planting and watching broccoli grow, and then eating it fresh from the plant, has revolutionized my attitude towards broccoli. I can now feed it to my baby with much more enthusiasm, which I'm sure he picks up. Knowing how to buy foods makes me very aware of how producers package food to get the attention of consumers. The concern for making money seems to be stronger than the concern for providing good nutritional quality to the public, in many instances. Selecting foods carefully can mean the difference between a wholesome, healthy diet and a low quality, unhealthy one. And Nikolas makes a "gagging-to-death" face when he gets canned baby food in his mouth!

. . .

FEEDING a young baby is very exciting. You may even find yourself eating foods and combinations of foods that you never considered before. You will find it helpful to have some basic cooking gear available, as well as a stock of healthy staple foods within easy reach so that your excitement can be based on knowledge and good nutrition.

Most parents have questions about their child's eating habits. The best general advice can be stated in one line: keep only healthy foods around the house. This way your children can eat anything they like while still getting something nutritious. If, from the very beginning, you don't stock the pantry with "junk" foods (and avoid exposing your child to too many advertisements and television commercials!), there will be fewer battles over eating habits, and if you do most of your shopping in natural food stores, many conflicts triggered by enticing supermarket displays will be prevented.[2] Even a one-year-old can be attracted by commercial displays. When sugar-coated cereals are not in sight, children cannot grab them off the shelves and are less likely to beg for them. If there are nuts, fruit, and whole foods treats by the checkout counter instead of stale, mass-market candy and gum, you will be less pressured to buy unwholesome snacks for the child who is crying while you are waiting in line to pay. It is much more satisfying to give your child a piece of fruit or a whole-grain fig cookie than a chocolate "zing" bar.

Variety is another way to keep your child content with eating healthy foods (although it might not seem that way when your child is going through a picky phase). Happily, a vegetarian diet is one of the most varied because of the huge number of different cultivated, edible plants that exist—literally thousands of varieties are grown around the world. If possible, try to grow at least some of your own food, a fascinating process that can entice your child to eat otherwise objectionable foods. The purchase of locally grown produce is another way to feel closer to the food you eat. Furthermore, there is a good chance that local farmers use fewer mass-production chemicals and techniques than do larger food companies, and if you patronize farmer's markets, you can ask the vendors about their growing practices.

A very interesting idea to think about is one presented by macrobiotic practitioners: people should try to eat foods which are in season. Most fruits and the more delicate vegetables, fresh from the garden, are eaten in the summer. Foods which can be stored, such as grains, beans, squashes, root vegetables, apples, and dried fruits, are eaten primarily in the winter. Even in the United States, most people follow a similar regimen at least part of the time; fruits and light salads are common summer meals, while heavier soups, stews, and baked goods are consumed during the winter, especially in regions where the weather is more extreme.

This macrobiotic principle of course should not be followed to such an extreme that your child does not obtain good nutrition all year round. The modern availability of fresh and frozen produce during even the darkest winter months can be a boon to parents trying to feed their children a well-rounded diet. But as Masanobu Fukuoka points out in his book, *The One-Straw Revolution:* "Compared with plants that ripen naturally . . . summer vegetables grown in the autumn or winter have none of the flavor and fragrance of those grown beneath the sun by organic and natural methods."[3] And since your child is unlikely to eat food that doesn't taste good, emphasizing properly grown foods in season is one way of ensuring a good intake of nutrients. The dearth of such foods in today's supermarkets probably accounts for many of the poor eating habits of modern Americans. Processed foods taste the same no matter what time of year, and the sugars, fats, and additives which they contain often have more flavor than most of the fruits and vegetables commonly available, even during the height of the growing season. Hard, anemic tomatoes and woody, bitter carrots just cannot compete with candy bars, ice cream, and sodas!

Finding basic vegetarian staples should present no problem in most cities. Rural dwellers can either make regular shopping trips to cities or order supplies from any of the major distributors of natural foods. A list of several such distributors is available in the Resource section.

Kitchen Tools

Remember, babies were eating mashed-up food from their parents' table long before prepared baby food was put into little jars![4]

Cost analyses show that making your own baby food is much cheaper than buying processed and packaged baby foods. Because fresh, high-quality ingredients can be used for homemade items, the nutritional value generally will be higher. Pre-prepared foods don't necessarily save much time. In fact, most meals made for a baby will take no more than five to ten minutes to prepare when starting from scratch. You will know exactly what is in each meal and probably will find your baby prefers homemade to canned baby foods.

The cost of equipping a kitchen for making vegetarian baby food does not have to be high. You probably already have most of the necessary items such as knives, forks, spoons, dishes, strainers, pots, and pans. You also probably own several kitchen appliances such as a blender, food processor, or juicer. Add a baby food grinder and bottle supplies, and you will be ready to go!

The following list of kitchen tools cannot possibly be comprehensive but is offered to give you ideas of what items you might want—if you don't already have them. Items that are useful for preparing meals for older children are included as well. Don't feel that you must have every one of these tools. Choose those that perform the functions you find most useful, and ignore the rest.

The Basics

Baby Food Grinder
This is the essential addition to a kitchen when a baby is born!

No electricity is needed, meal-size proportions are easily made, an ideal consistency is produced—all for only a few dollars compared to more elaborate appliances. Baby food grinders are available at general department stores across the country, and in many kitchen stores and grocery stores, as well.

The baby food grinder is a simplified version of a food mill. Any food that has been partially cooked or is naturally soft can be put into the grinder. After fitting the grinding arm and sieve into place, you grind while pushing down, and soon the freshly ground meal comes out the top ready to eat. The food can then be scraped into a bowl from which to feed your baby, although it is also possible to spoon the food directly from the top dish of the grinder. This wonderful appliance can be used for the "fast-food" recipes given in chapter six or for transforming adult meals into purées. The grinder prepares enough food for one or two meals at a time, depending upon how much your baby eats.

Bottles and Bottle Supplies

A good supply of bottles is obviously a necessity for the bottle-fed baby, but even breast-fed babies may occasionally need to use one. Bottles come in many different sizes and styles, such as eight-ounce glass bottles, smaller glass bottles, plastic bottles, bottles with bags which reduce the amount of air your baby swallows, clear bottles, decorated bottles, and so on. Different nipples also are available, such as milk nipples and juice nipples. Buy whatever makes you and your baby happy.

A bottle-cleaning brush is essential because there is no other way to get the milk film off the inside of the bottle when hand-washing, especially if the used bottle sits for any length of time. Cleaning bottles is very, very important, especially during the first six months of your baby's life. Most people recommend boiling bottles and nipples at least once in a while to get rid of all the bacteria. But when hand-washing, use water that is as hot as you can stand, scrub well with the brush and soap, and rinse thoroughly. It is as important to get all the soap out as it is to get the bottle clean. Of course, a good quality dishwasher is even better at getting bottles really clean.

Pots and Pans

Small pots and pans are ideal for food preparation for very young babies. Large pots and pans can be used to make enough for the whole family, including leftovers for refrigerating or freezing to get you through the week.

Knives

A good, sharp knife is very important for preparing foods. The more finely a food is chopped, the more quickly it will cook. A knife is also good for making bite-size pieces of fruits, vegetables, and breads for older babies. Invest in the highest quality knives you can afford and, for an initial set, start with paring, six to eight-inch chef's, and bread knives. If you also purchase a sharpening stone and wood block, and learn to care for and store your knives properly, they will last a lifetime. When working with and storing knives, be especially careful to keep them out of the reach of a toddler!

Baby Spoons

Baby spoons are smaller than adult spoons and fit into a baby's mouth more easily. They also hold less food so that you are less likely to put more into your baby's mouth than he or she can handle at one time. There are spoons with curved handles (easier for the baby to hold, without the danger of a poke in the eye) and with straight handles. There are plastic spoons and metal spoons. Choose whatever you find most convenient.

Baby Cups

As you wean your baby, you may find a baby cup (or two or three) to be useful. These cups are small, plastic, and come with special "sipper" lids or straws that children enjoy using; their prevention of spills appeals to parents! You also will want your child to learn to use a regular cup, but sometimes a baby cup is just the thing.

Potato Masher

A potato masher can be used to crush soft foods, especially well-cooked root vegetables. They also work well to mash tofu and beans for sandwich fillings.

Grater

A grater is a wonderful device to get vegetables to a quick-cooking stage that matches the short time needed to cook pre-ground grains and legumes. The large round holes work the best. Graters come in many shapes and sizes. You might want both a stand-up grater and a flat one which can be laid across a bowl.

Strainer

A mesh strainer can help make fruit and vegetable juices fine enough to be sucked through a nipple. Strain items more than once or use a strainer with a very fine mesh. When your child is older, straining certain foods can reduce the chance of the child choking on unexpected lumps in otherwise smooth foods.

Vegetable Scrubbers, Peelers, and Soaps

Scrubbers are great for cleaning dirt, chemicals, and fertilizers (including organic ones) from hard fruits and vegetables. According to the FDA, washing produce with soap is not necessary, but a squirt of vegetable-based dish soap or specialty produce soap, followed by a good rinse, certainly won't hurt most produce either. Use it if it makes you feel more comfortable. Peeling is a viable alternative to washing in many cases, especially for babies. Clean peels can be stored in the refrigerator and used to make broth.

Other Useful Tools

Multi-Purpose Slicing Tool

When your child is able to eat raw, crunchy vegetables, you can use one of these "slicing, dicing" tools to quickly cut them into a variety of interesting shapes.

Food Mill

A good food mill will grind up whole grains into smaller grains, flours, or powders, depending upon the tightness of the grinder and the number of times you run the grain through. You can use a food mill once every month or two, each time grinding up a supply of grains and legumes into a rough powder (one time through) and storing them in capped glass jars in the refrigerator. These ground-up foods keep like flours and can be used to make main dishes within minutes. Simply add three parts water to one part powder. Cook grains until they are soft; cook most legumes for at least ten minutes and soybeans for twenty. (*See Legumes, page 170.*) The three-to-one ratio depends on the temperature at which you cook the grain, so experiment—but keep an eye on it, because it cooks fast.

Food mills also can be used to grind up nuts and seeds to make butters. Nothing else needs to be added because of the natural oils already present. Don't make large quantities of nut and seed butters, however, as the fats in nuts and seeds can become rancid quickly (*see Storage and Handling, below*).

Blenders, Grinders, Food Processors, and Juicers

You probably already own at least one of these appliances. Each appliance has a slightly different function, although there is some overlap.

Blenders make good fruit drinks, smoothies, and blended soups. Hand blenders are especially useful for the latter as they can be used right in the cooking pot. Blenders also can be used to powder small amounts of nuts and seeds, including flax seeds if water is added. And at least one blender (the Vita-Mix) can be used to cook or freeze foods as they are blended.

Small coffee-style grinders can be used to powder nuts, seeds, and spices. (If you drink coffee, buy two—one for coffee beans, and the other for everything else.) You won't produce a nut butter this way, but coarsely ground nuts and seeds can be used in many dishes, and a grinder is easy to use when just a tablespoon or so is needed.

Food processors are multi-purpose machines which can grind, blend, chop, grate, and mix a multitude of foods. They come in many different sizes. You might find the smallest size to be just right for baby foods while a large size can be used for family meals.

Juicers are used to make fresh fruit and vegetable juices and sauces from raw produce. While you won't want to give a child too much juice, several ounces a week can be a healthful way to assure that your child is getting enough vitamins and minerals. Fruit juices, and fruit or vegetable purées, can be used in baked goods, and vegetable juices can be cooked into grains or used as a base in soups. Some juicers come with a grain attachment that can be used like a food mill.

Rice Cookers, Bread Bakers, and Pressure Cookers

This trio of kitchen tools can greatly assist the whole foods cook who is short of time. You will have to experiment to learn how best to use them, but once you do, you will never look back. Make sure you buy items that are designed to handle whole grains. Modern pressure cookers come with multiple safety devices, so if you have an old and not-so-safe pressure cooker, this is a good time to invest in a new one.

Crock Pots, Clay Pots

If you prefer to slow-cook foods, crock pots for the stove and clay pots for the oven can be a good investment. They have the advantage of fully developing the flavors of foods while retaining nutrients and increasing digestibility.

Toasters and Toaster Ovens

Older children are sure to appreciate toast, waffles, and other items that can easily be prepared in these appliances. Compared to the regular oven, a toaster oven can save fuel when small quantities of foods are being reheated or cooked. As for regular toasters, those with wide slots designed for foods like bagels are the most versatile.

Microwave Oven

A microwave can greatly speed up many cooking processes, and they are safe so long as they are maintained and used properly. Just make sure to test the temperature of any food you heat in a microwave very carefully before giving it to your baby because the inside of the food can become *extremely* hot in a very short time, even if the outside still feels relatively cool. For this reason, liquids such as formula should not be heated in a microwave.

Yogurt Maker

Commercially made yogurt makers all have one thing in common: an electrically heated base that keeps the yogurt at the proper temperature. They vary in details like covers and timers and the design of the yogurt containers. You can easily make yogurt without a yogurt maker; the advantage it offers is the steady temperature, which consistently produces smooth-textured yogurt.

Although yogurt is readily available at the store, few brands use organic ingredients, and most contain large amounts of sweeteners. By making your own yogurt, you have control over the ingredients. Another plus is the ability to make non-dairy yogurts, which can be difficult to find commercially.

Food Selection, Storage, and Handling

Such a wide variety of grains, legumes, fresh produce, and other vegetarian food is available that it is impossible to cover everything completely in one book, but this section contains the basics on the selection, storage, and handling of some of the more common, easily digested, and easily prepared foods. For quick reference, Table 5.1 (*below*) lists the different categories of whole foods, the major nutrients found in each, and the basic directions for preparing each type of food for a baby or young child.

Table 5.1: (Selected) Foods, Nutrition and Preparation

Type of Food	Nutrition Information	Preparation
Grains		
brown rice millet barley lentils breads & cereals oatmeal	B vitamins, vitamin E zinc, copper, iron, magnesium, phosphorus, carbohydrates fats protein, *especially when combined with legumes, seeds or dairy products*	1. Grind up dry grain in fine food mill until a rough powdery consistency is reached. 2. Cook three parts water to one part grain until pasty consistency is reached. Cool and season (optional) and serve. 3. Store extra in closed container in refrigerator.
Legumes		
soybeans mung beans lentils split peas chick peas	same as grains protein, *especially when combined with grains or nuts and seeds*	1. Same as for grains 2. Cook in three to four parts water for ten to fifteen minutes. (Soybeans for twenty minutes.) 3. Same as for grains
Vegetables		
broccoli cabbage spinach carrots squash sweet potatoes oeas lima beans	*green vegetables* calcium, copper, vitamin B-2, vitamin C, folacin *yellow vegetables* chromium, vitamins A & C	*(for cooked vegetables only)* 1. Cut into thin slices 2. Cook in small amount of water at low temperature or add extra water to grains and cook with grains until water is gone. 3. Blend through baby food grinder or serve in chunks as baby requests.
Nuts & Seeds		
almonds sesame seeds brazil nuts cashews	same as grains protein, *especially when combined with grains, legumes*	1. Grind through food mill until the consistency of pasty butter. 2. Mix with legumes or rice or serve as nut balls. 3. Eat **immediately**: Does not store well over long periods.
Fruits		
dried fruits figs, dates, raisins, apricots, prunes *fresh fruits* bananas, apples, pears, coconut	natural sweeteners B vitamins, vitamins A & C calcium, chromium, iron	*dried fruits:* Soak in water until plump, or add small chunks to grain while cooking.Use baby food grinder to blend into food. Can also be eaten raw by older children. *fresh fruits:* Don't cook! Mash with fork or baby food grinder or give as finger foods to older babies.

Grains

As is true for adults, a child's diet should be based on grains.

The Vegetarian Way[5]

Most food grains are the seeds of grasses with some coming from non-grass plants. Each seed is made of three parts. The germ, or heart of the seed, is particularly high in B-complex vitamins, vitamin E, iron, protein, and carbohydrates. Covering the germ is the endosperm, which is the largest part of the grain and primarily carbohydrate with traces of minerals and vitamins. The bran is the outer covering, providing fiber along with traces of minerals (especially iron), B-complex vitamins, and some amino acids. Products made from whole grains generally are preferable to those made from refined grains because B-complex vitamins, vitamin E, fiber, and iron are lost during the milling process, but children generally can benefit from the extra calories provided by reasonable amounts of less-fibrous processed grains in items such as pasta, couscous, and cold cereals, especially if fortified products are used.

Purchase only the freshest whole grains. Stale grain will smell musty or moldy and may have evidence of insect infestation. To ensure that the grains you buy are as fresh as possible, purchase them from a reputable mail order company or a food store that practices good hygiene and has fast turnover of their bulk products. Only buy what your family will use within a few months. When you get the grain home, store it in a tightly capped, glass jar in a cool, dark place. The refrigerator or freezer are ideal, especially for milled products such as flours, as they will inhibit oxidation (rancidity) of the oils present in the grain. Whole grains also can be frozen for 24 hours to kill insect eggs before storage elsewhere.

The most commonly used grains are rice, oats, corn, wheat, barley, and rye. Other grains your baby might enjoy include amaranth, quinoa, millet, buckwheat, spelt, Kamut, and triticale. You will find a list below which details the special strengths of each, but all grains are important sources of protein, iron, and B vitamins and so, very important for the growing baby. Grains are commonly one of the first solid foods fed to a baby, but some parents choose to wait until after the introduction of fruits and vegetables, especially if there is a family history of allergy. The first grains to be introduced should be non-glutinous grains such as brown rice, millet, and quinoa, followed by barley and oats, and finally corn and wheat which are the hardest grains to digest and most likely to be allergy-forming, especially if given to a child under 12 months of age.

The important thing to remember is that the grains must be cooked thoroughly for the young baby in order to ease digestion. Preparing grain either can be done by cooking it first and then grinding it through a baby food grinder to make it into a smooth paste, or by grinding the fresh grain into a powder with a food mill or grain grinder and then cooking it as needed. Blend the grain with a caloric liquid—breast milk or formula to start with; other liquids as the child can tolerate them—for a smooth, moist texture which is dilute enough for a baby to swallow easily. Feed the grain to the baby with a spoon—never put cereal, however dilute, into a bottle!

Amaranth

This very small grain-like seed was eaten originally by the Aztecs (the leaves also are highly nutritious). Amaranth contains a large amount of protein, calcium, and iron as well as vitamin C. It can be used to make a rather gelatinous hot cereal, is excellent when mixed with other flours in baked goods, and can be puffed like popcorn or sprouted like alfalfa.

Barley

Barley is a good winter grain since it tends to be more filling than other grains. It is fairly easy to digest and is a good source of niacin, thiamin, and trace minerals. Hulled barley is the least processed, pearled barley is the most processed, and Scotch barley is in between. Cook barley as you would rice, add it to soups and salads, or use it as a hot cereal. You also might want to try malted barley syrup, a flavorful sweetener, with a texture similar to honey, which is made from sprouted, toasted whole barley.

Buckwheat

Buckwheat is another seed which is eaten like a grain. It is an excellent source of B-complex vitamins, calcium, and phosphorus. Buckwheat groats make an excellent hot cereal, and buckwheat flour is a wonderful addition to other flours in baked goods such as pancakes.

Corn

Corn originated in Central and South America several thousand years ago where peoples such as the Incas began to breed large ears from small, wild seed heads. Fresh corn is used as a vegetable, but dried corn is eaten as a grain. Corn supplies B-complex vitamins and large quantities of vitamin A, with blue corn being higher in protein than yellow corn. Dried kernels can be soaked and added to soups and casseroles. Cornmeal makes an excellent hot cereal (mush or polenta) and can be used to make baked goods such as corn bread. Corn flours are the basis for items such as tortillas, tamales, cold cereals, and chips. Look for tortillas made with lime as the calcium will be more available. Popcorn is a wonderful vehicle for nutritional yeast, and children adore it, but it can be a choking hazard for babies and toddlers. Dr. Spock suggests feeding foods like popcorn only to children who are calmly sitting at a table while under adult supervision.[6]

Kamut®

Kamut (pronounced "kah-moot´") is the brand name of an ancient variety of wheat which is high in protein, vitamin E, and minerals. Some people who are allergic to modern wheat can eat Kamut.

Millet

This small, round grain contains plentiful amounts of protein, B-complex vitamins, calcium, and iron. Its lack of gluten makes it as easy to digest as rice, so millet cereal is an excellent early food for babies. Later, whole millet can be baked into bread or cooked with other grains, and the flour can be added to other grains in baked goods such as muffins.

Oats

Oats have a high protein and iron content as well as B-complex vitamins, calcium, magnesium, and other nutrients. Oats are most commonly rolled and served as hot oatmeal cereal, but whole oats are excellent when cooked with rice and other grains, and oat flour is wonderful when added to other grains in baked goods.

Quinoa

This small grain (pronounced "keen´-wa") originated with the Incas of Peru, and it is exceptionally high in good-quality protein as well as containing appreciable amounts of fat, B-complex vitamins, vitamin E, iron, calcium, and phosphorus. Quinoa has a coating of bitter saponin which must be thoroughly washed off before cooking—rinse under running water until the water runs clear. It cooks very quickly and is not glutinous which makes it an excellent baby food.

Rice

By using the many varieties of rice available today, you can add interest to your child's diet. Babies do very well starting with fortified rice cereals which are easy to digest and supply B vitamins, calcium, phosphorus, and iron. Older children might enjoy arborio, basmati, japonica, and jasmine rices in addition to the usual long, medium, and short grain white or brown rices. Rice is used by itself and as a component of a variety of dishes such as soups, salads, and desserts. It also can be made into beverages (rice milk, amazake) and the Japanese treat, mochi, all of which are very popular with children due to their sweet taste.

Rye

Rye contains high levels of protein, B-complex vitamins, iron, and calcium, with dark rye containing more nutrients than light rye. Whole rye berries have a very strong flavor which is best when mixed with milder grains such as rice. Rye bread and hot rye cereal are also good.

Spelt

Like Kamut, spelt is a wheat relative which often can be eaten by people who suffer from allergies. Spelt is available commercially as whole berries and flour as well as in products such as pasta, bread, and cereals.

Teff

Teff is an extremely small, non-glutinous grain which is exceptionally high in iron as well as protein, thiamin, and calcium. It comes in three colors: red, white, and brown. The whole grain makes a good hot cereal while teff flour is an excellent addition to baked goods such as pancakes and muffins, and is used to make the Ethiopian bread, injera.

Triticale

This grain (pronounced "tri-ti-kay´-lee") is a rye-wheat hybrid which contains a large amount of protein. It is available whole as well as in the form of flakes and flour and can be used in the same fashion as wheat and rye. Like wheat, it can contribute to allergies and so should not be fed to babies younger than 12 months.

Wheat

Wheat is high in protein, B-complex vitamins, iron, and calcium. Because of its high gluten content, it is less easily digested than other grains and so shouldn't be fed until your baby is at least 12 months old. Wheat is very versatile and comes in many forms, including whole berries, flakes, flours, couscous, and bulgur. Wheat germ and wheat bran are byproducts of the refining process in the manufacture of white flour. Wheat germ is very nutritious and can be a delicious addition to baked goods, but it should not be considered a substitute for whole grains. Wheat bran can lead to too much phytic acid and fiber in the diet of a young child and so should not be added to your child's food. Seitan is a product made from wheat gluten which is very high in protein and is used as a meat substitute. Because of its extremely high gluten content (nearly 100 percent), it should only be fed in small amounts to older children who tolerate gluten well.

Wild Rice

This seed of a North American grass is not a true rice but is used in much the same way. Because it has a strong flavor, most people prefer it when mixed with other grains. It also can be popped like popcorn or ground into flour for use in baked goods.

RESOURCES

The New Book of Whole Grains: More Than 200 Recipes Featuring Whole Grains, Including Amaranth, Quinoa, Wheat, Spelt, Oats, Rye, Barley, and Millet by Marlene Anne Bumilligramsarner and Johanna Roy, illustrator (St. Martin's Griffin, 1997).

Amazing Grains: Creating Vegetarian Main Dishes with Whole Grains by Joanne Saltzman (H J Kramer, 1990).

Legumes

First protein foods for vegetarian infants can be thoroughly cooked and puréed legumes or well-mashed tofu.[7]

Legume is a general term which includes beans, dried peas, and lentils. Like grains, legumes are seeds, but they are found enclosed within pods. Legumes are a major source of carbohydrates, proteins, and fiber, and they also contain significant amounts of iron, calcium, thiamin, riboflavin and niacin. When sprouted, legumes provide vitamin C.

Only fresh and clean legumes should be purchased, and they should be stored in glass jars in a cool, dry place. Whole, dry legumes can be stored in a cupboard, but if you grind dry or sprouted legumes, you will want to put them in the refrigerator. Before use, wash legumes well, and carefully discard discolored and broken seeds along with any small rocks or other debris.

Since legumes are harder to digest than grains, they should be added to your child's diet somewhat later, preferably after seven to eight months. The Farm community suggests that split pea soup be one of the first legume foods introduced to the baby. The most important thing to remember when feeding legumes to babies is to cook the legumes very, very well. With longer cooking times, the legume is more easily digested, resulting in less gas. Also, the trypsin inhibitor, which is found in some legumes such as soybeans and can interfere with protein digestion, is broken down by longer cooking.

Ideally, legumes to be used for baby food should be soaked for 12 to 24 hours. The soaking water should then be poured off and replaced with clean water before gently simmering the legumes for several hours until they are very soft. If you haven't the time for long cooking, a pressure cooker can accomplish the same thing much more quickly. Many beans also are available canned. Look for organic varieties, and rinse them before using. The cooked legumes should be put through a baby food grinder and then sieved to remove any husks or skins, which are hard to digest.

Another technique is to grind dried legumes into a powder much like grains, and to store this powder in airtight containers in the refrigerator to have on hand for quicker cooking. Quicker cooking in this case means ten to 15 minutes for most legumes and 20 minutes for soybeans.

Any legume can be sprouted simply by modifying the soaking process. One study of mung beans found that sprouting decreased unwanted substances like phytic acid, tannin, and raffinose, while increasing important nutrients such as glucose, folic acid, and vitamin C, and making the iron and protein more bioavailable.[8] To sprout legumes, place them in a clean glass jar or special sprouting tray, cover them with water, and soak them overnight. The next morning, rinse the legumes and then continue to rinse them two or three times a day for three or four days until the sprouted portion is the same length as the original seed. Discard any unsprouted seeds. If using a jar, cover it with a paper towel and rubber band or a fine screen to help conserve moisture but to allow fresh air in so the legumes do not rot or develop mold. Certain varieties of legume sprouts can be used raw by adults, but given the possibility of contamination (especially if store-bought) and the difficulty of cleaning, they probably should not be fed to a young child. Other sprouts, such as soybeans and kidney beans, need to be cooked which should reduce or eliminate any contamination problems.

Some legumes are processed extensively in order to make them more digestible. Soybeans are the prime example: tofu is an extremely digestible processed form of this legume with very high protein, fat, calcium, iron, phosphorus, potassium, sodium, B vitamins, choline, and vitamin E content.

Soybeans and soy products are nutritional powerhouses that are often the basis of commercial faux-meat products. Tofu, soy milk, and soy yogurt can be introduced into the baby's diet at about seven or eight months of age, although families with a history of allergies would be wise to wait until the baby is a full year old as soy is a common allergen. Also, please note that although the soybeans are cooked in the making of tofu, the tofu itself is similar to a raw product that can develop molds or become contaminated by improper handling. Buy tofu in packages rather than from open tubs, store it in the refrigerator, and change the water daily after opening. Before use, rinse tofu well to remove any surface bacteria. You also can steam it for several minutes. Throw out any tofu that develops an odor or visible mold.

Hundreds of varieties of legumes with different shapes, sizes, colors, flavors, and textures, are available from heirloom growers. While natural food stores sometimes carry several types of legumes, mail order companies offer many, many more. (*See Resources, page 247, for information on suppliers.*) Because of the large number of available legumes, it is impossible to discuss them all, but the following list includes the basics. Many vegetarian cookbooks contain sections on beans, but for more information a good bean cookbook can be invaluable.

Adzuki Beans

The adzuki is mostly used in Japanese, Chinese, and macrobiotic dishes. The adzuki can be used like any other bean but often is mashed into a paste with additional flavorings. When mixed with sugar, it is used for Asian desserts such as red bean cakes. Raw adzuki bean sprouts also can be ground into a flour which can be added to baked goods.

Black Beans

Black beans are a major component of Mexican and South Western cooking, and they are high in calcium, potassium, and phosphorus. They commonly are cooked into soups, used whole in salads or burritos, and mashed or refried for use as a dip or spread.

Black-eyed Peas

These are great for quick meals as they needn't be soaked before cooking. With a pressure cooker, you can go from dried to cooked black-eyed peas in approximately ten to 20 minutes!

Chickpeas

Also called garbanzo beans, this legume is a staple of the Middle East where it is used to make hummus and falafel, foods which are very popular with vegetarian children. Chickpeas and chickpea flour also are used in East Indian cooking, especially curries and breads.

Dried Peas

When fresh, peas are eaten as a vegetable, but dried green and yellow peas, either split or whole, make wonderful soups, dips, spreads, and pilafs which are very digestible for babies and young children.

Fava Beans

This bean is known by many names such as broad bean, horse bean, and Scotch bean. Favas are a very large bean which many people like to use in heavier foods such as soups or stews. Some people (most commonly males with African or Mediterranean ancestry) have a rather rare genetic predisposition to a condition called favism which creates an acute anemia upon consumption of fava beans, so if you feed these beans to your child, watch for any adverse reactions.

Lentils

Green, brown, red, and yellow lentils are commonly used in East Indian cooking, in dishes such as dal. They can be used in soups, salads, pilafs, and spreads and also are an excellent meat substitute in foods such as burgers and loafs. Lentils are a great baby food as they rarely cause allergies, need not be soaked before cooking, and when boiled, form a rich broth that needs no additions. Lentils also are suitable for use as sprouts.

Kidney Beans

Bean chili and bean salads are the dishes in which kidney beans are most used. Kidney beans should always be cooked before eating.

Lima Beans

Also called butter beans, lima beans are one of the most popular legumes in the United States. These large, white beans are good in soups, salads, stews, and casseroles, and also can be mashed to form a spread or side dish.

Mung Beans

Like adzuki beans, mung beans are a popular Asian food. They are very small, green beans which generally are sprouted and used raw in salads or cooked in stir-fries. They also can be used in soups and other foods. Because they are so small, they cook relatively quickly and, therefore, make an excellent addition to a grain pilaf.

Pinto Beans

Like black beans, pinto beans are used in Mexican cuisine. Refried beans are usually made from pinto beans, and children love them spread on tortillas. The whole beans are excellent in soups and other dishes.

Soy Beans

As mentioned above, soybeans are extremely versatile and have become a mainstay of vegetarian cuisine due to their high nutritional content and malleability. Soybeans can be used as other beans, but they also can be turned into flour, grits, textured vegetable protein (TVP), tempeh, tofu, silken tofu, miso, yuba, soy sauce, soy milk, soy yogurt, soy cheese, and soy ice cream. The following books contain detailed information on the many uses of soybeans.

RESOURCES

Lean Bean Cuisine: Over 100 Tasty Meatless Recipes from Around the World by Jay Solomon (Prima Publishing, 1994).

Calypso Bean Soup: And Other Savory Recipes Featuring Heirloom Beans from the West by Lesa Heebner (Harper-Collins, 1996). This book contains a few non-vegetarian recipes but is unique in its focus on heirloom beans.

The Book of Tofu: Protein Source of the Future—Now by William Shurtleff and Akiko Aoyagi (Celestial Arts, 1998).

The Book of Miso by William Shurtleff and Akiko Aoyagi (Ballantine Books, 1989).

New Soy Cookbook: Tempting Recipes for Soybeans, Soy Milk, Tofu, Tempeh, Miso and Soy Sauce by Lorna J. Sass (Chronicle Books, 1998). This book includes some seafood recipes but has many recipes and ideas suitable for vegetarians.

Nuts and Seeds

Nuts from trees, and some seeds from plants, are very high in healthy fats and fat-soluble vitamin E as well as protein, fiber, iron, calcium, and other vitamins and minerals. Buy small quantities of fresh, whole nuts, preferably organically grown and in the shell. Because of their high fat content, nuts and seeds rapidly go rancid when shelled, chopped, or made into butters and oils. Store seeds, shelled nuts, and products made from them in glass jars in the refrigerator or freezer, and throw them out if they develop a disagreeable odor. Foods prepared with nut and seed products should be treated similarly. Nuts still in their shells can be stored loosely in porous bags such as burlap in a dark, cool, dry place.

Nuts and seeds in their natural form are not digestible by babies, and they can be contaminated with an aflatoxin-producing fungus that is potentially very harmful to young children. In addition, whole nuts and seeds, and sticky nut butters such as peanut butter, can be a choking hazard. Most seed foods, therefore, should not be introduced until near the end of the first year, and nut foods only after 12 months. The introduction of whole nuts and seeds should wait until the child is three to four years old and safely able to chew them.

Although not a substitute for breast milk or formula, delicious nut and seed milks can be a high-energy addition to a toddler's diet. Almond milk is available commercially, but to make other nut and seed milks, soak the nuts or seeds in the refrigerator overnight, and then blend them into the soaking liquid. The blending has to be done in a food processor or good quality blender, and the food must then be strained to remove any small chunks. Add fruit, sweeteners, and other ingredients for interest and increased nutrition. If you want more ideas, a great recipe book is available: *Not Milk . . . Nut Milks: 40 of the Most Original Dairy-Free Recipes Ever* by Candia Lea Cole (Woodbridge Press, 1997).

You also can make a type of yogurt from nuts and seeds rather than from a milk base. Steve Meyerowitz, in the August, 1979 issue of *Vegetarian Times*, offers the following recipe:

> Soak sesame seeds, sunflower seeds, cashews or almonds overnight and sprout for one day if you wish (sprouting is optional). Blend with 3 parts water for yoghurt. Place in warm area, 80 to 100° Fahrenheit for 8 hours with a loose cover. Rising and the presence of air bubbles indicate it is ready. The taste should be tart and sour. You can strain off the liquid and drink it. The strained pulp is your cheese or yoghurt.[9]

Almonds

Almonds are actually a fruit kernel related to peaches, which is easy to see when you buy them in the shell. They can be eaten raw, toasted, blanched, or as a butter. As noted above, commercial almond milk is readily available, or it can be made at home. Grinding almonds produces a meal or flour which can be added to baked goods for an especially delicious and delicate flavor and texture.

Brazil Nuts

Brazils are very large nuts which can be chopped and added to a variety of dishes, or ground into a nut butter.

Cashews

Each fruit of the cashew tree develops a single cashew nut at the end. The shells contain a caustic substance that must be removed during processing so they cannot be bought in the shell. Cashews are wonderful raw or dry-roasted, added to stir-fries, made into a milk or butter, or blended with other ingredients such as silken tofu, sugar, and vanilla extract to form a cream to be used on desserts.

Chestnuts

The only low-fat nut, chestnuts are wonderfully sweet which makes them great for dessert recipes. While they can be eaten raw, they are best when roasted. Bottled chestnuts are available for use in recipes when cooking and peeling them yourself is too difficult.

Coconut

Although very high in saturated fat, a small amount of coconut is an acceptable part of most vegetarian diets, and most children love it—especially if they get to help open a fresh nut! The flesh is a great snack or addition to baked goods while the milk can be used in recipes such as curries, stir-fries, and rice puddings. When buying commercially prepared coconut, look for unsweetened, unsulfured products.

Flax Seeds

Flax is one of the best plant sources of omega-3 fatty acids and, therefore, belongs in every vegetarian kitchen although it should not be used to the exclusion of other seeds, nuts, and oils. Whole flax tends not to digest well, even in adults, so briefly grind the seeds before using them in soups, cereals, and breads. You also can blend ground flax seeds with water to use as a binder in baked goods. Flax goes rancid extremely quickly, so buy small quantities from a good supplier, freeze or refrigerate them, and use them within a short time.

Hazelnuts

These nuts grow on shrubs. (Filberts are a similar nut which are produced by a tree.) They are great for stuffing vegetables like squashes and also can be roasted and ground into a butter.

Macadamia Nuts

Macadamia nuts are delicious, but because of their high saturated fat content, they are best used in small quantities. A commercial macadamia nut butter is available or you can make your own. Sliced macadamia nuts are good in salads or on fruit.

Peanuts

Also called ground-nuts, peanuts are actually a legume, but because of their high fat content they are classified as a nut by nutritionists. Because they can be a potent allergen, a choking hazard, and often are contaminated with aflatoxin fungi, peanuts and peanut butter should be among the last foods to be introduced to your child, which is ironic given how closely peanut butter is associated with vegetarian diets! Peanuts are delicious, however, and peanut butter is readily available in many restaurants and homes, so go ahead and introduce them to your child somewhere between 18 and 24 months unless an allergic reaction develops.

Pecans

Pecans are from a North American tree related to the hickory.

They can be used in essentially every type of dish and are especially delicious when roasted.

Pine Nuts

Although called nuts, pine nuts are the seeds of various pine trees such as the piñon pine. They taste best if lightly roasted before use. Due to their high oil content and tendency to turn rancid, they are best bought in small quantities and used quickly. Spanish pignolias are a type of pine nut with somewhat less fat and considerably more protein than the American ones.

Pistachio Nuts

Avoid artificially dyed pistachios. Eat pistachios raw or roasted, and use them in rice pudding and nut bread.

Pumpkin Seeds

One of the most nutritious seeds, pumpkin seeds are very popular with children, especially when home-roasted after making a jack-o'-lantern at Halloween! Some other winter squash seeds can be treated similarly.

Sesame Seeds

Like flax, sesame seeds are difficult to digest when whole, but calcium-rich sesame seed butter and tahini, either toasted or raw, are excellent foods for young children. Use them to thicken soups and to spread on breads and crackers. Or make the delicious sesame-based candy, halvah, for your toddler.

Sunflower Seeds

Sunflower seeds are extremely nutritious. Use sunflower seeds to make luscious butters, milks, and sprouts. Sunflowers come in many varieties and are fun to grow and shell, so they are a great plant for a child's garden.

Walnuts

This popular nut is a good source of omega-3 fatty acid and can be added to almost any dish from oatmeal to salad to casseroles. If you buy walnuts in the shell, consider getting a shelling device which doesn't destroy the hulls as they can be used in craft projects.

Vegetables

Vegetables are the roots, stems, leaves, shoots, flowers, and sometimes fruits of plants. In general, vegetables are very low in fat while providing carbohydrates and water along with vitamin A, vitamin C, potassium, and fiber. Certain types of vegetables also contain significant amounts of protein, B vitamins, calcium, iron, magnesium, and trace minerals. In addition to nutrients, vegetables add texture, variety, and color to a meal. They often are divided into groups by their color, which can indicate both their nutritional makeup and their culinary use. Common groups are light green, dark green, and yellow/orange.

Light green vegetables provide vitamins, minerals, and fiber. They include celery, cabbage, and cauliflower. Yellow/orange and dark green vegetables are the best sources of carotenes and vitamin C. Yellow/orange vegetables also contain the trace mineral chromium. The leafy dark green vegetables are very nutritious, containing calcium, B vitamins (especially folacin, often missing in the American diet), and iron. In general, the darker green the leaf, the richer it will be in minerals and vitamins. Broccoli, for example, is one of the highest sources of vitamin C, calcium, and riboflavin, the B vitamin most commonly deficient in the American diet. Another leafy green, kale, is one of the best dietary sources of calcium.

Look carefully at vegetables before you buy them. Leafy vegetables should be crisp and fresh; brown or dark spots indicate that decay has started at which point they should not be fed to a baby. Other vegetables should be firm and unbruised. Wash all vegetables when you are ready to eat them and not before; leafy vegetables in particular are usually damaged by washing and should, therefore, be eaten immediately before damage turns to decay. Most fresh vegetables should be stored in sealed plastic bags in the refrigerator, but winter squashes and some root vegetables such as potatoes can be stored in a cool, dark place such as a cupboard or root cellar. If potatoes begin to sprout or turn green, you won't want to feed them to your baby, but you can cut away the bad spots and use them for yourself.

When preparing vegetables for young babies, it is necessary to cook them until they are soft, which unfortunately destroys the vitamin C content to a great extent. Also, much of the mineral and water-soluble vitamin content is lost into the cooking water. To minimize this loss, cut the vegetable into very thin slices or small cubes right before cooking, and then cook them quickly in as little water as possible (you can always add more). If you cook vegetables and grains simultaneously in the same pot, you will not waste any of the water because it will be absorbed into the grain. If you cook the vegetables separately, cook them first with only a little water, and then use the leftover nutrient-rich water when cooking grains and legumes, or when making broth.

As your child develops teeth and becomes adept at chewing, you can begin to offer more lightly cooked and less processed vegetables. Cut or slice them to an appropriate size, and only feed them to your child when he or she is sitting quietly at a table while under direct adult supervision. The American Academy of Pediatrics suggests delaying the introduction of raw vegetables until three years as they are a major choking hazard.[10] You probably won't want to wait that long, but you will want to be extra vigilant when feeding raw, crunchy vegetables such as carrots to a toddler.

So many varieties and types of vegetables exist that it is impossible to list more than a few of them. The following vegetables have excellent nutritional value, and are often a favorite with babies and toddlers: asparagus, artichoke hearts, beets, broccoli, Brussels sprouts, cabbage, carrots, cauliflower, collards, cucumbers, eggplant, fresh corn, fresh Lima beans, fresh peas, jicama, kale, lettuces, mushrooms, okra, parsley, parsnips, plantains, potatoes, radishes, rutabagas, spinach, sweet peppers, sweet potatoes, tomatoes, turnips, winter squashes, zucchini. Details on a few of the most common vegetables are listed below.

Beets

This plant is grown for both the roots and greens. The roots are best when baked whole in the same manner as a potato. They also are great in soups such as the classic borsht. The greens are eaten raw, or are steamed or stir-fried like other leafy vegetables. Both roots and greens contain fiber, carotenes, B-complex vitamins, vitamin C, calcium, iron, magnesium, phosphorus, and potassium.

Broccoli

Broccoli is a member of the cruciferous family, which also contains Brussels sprouts, cabbage, cauliflower, and similar vegetables. Both peeled stems and florets can be eaten raw, but generally the florets are best when cooked through blanching, steaming, or stir-frying. Broccoli contains protein, fiber, carotenes, B-complex vitamins, vitamin C, calcium, phosphorus, and potassium.

Carrots

One of the most popular vegetables, carrots are packed with carotenes. They also contain other nutrients such as fiber, calcium, and potassium. Carrots should be cooked for young children, but older children will enjoy them either cooked or raw. Use them by themselves or in soups, stews, salads, juices, and baked goods.

Kale

Another member of the cruciferous family, kale is one of the most nutritious greens, being one of the best plant sources of calcium. Shredded raw kale can be used in salads, but it is best when steamed or stir-fried.

Mushrooms

These fungi come in a large variety of colors, flavors, and textures which can add a "meaty" component to many dishes. Try chanterelles, crimini, enoki, morel, oyster, portobello, and shiitake mushrooms in addition to the more common button mushroom. Use them raw in salads or cooked in a variety of dishes such as soups, stir-fries, and gravies. Nutritionally, mushrooms contain protein, biotin, calcium, iron, phosphorus, potassium, and trace amounts of other minerals.

Peas

Fresh green peas are a favorite of babies! Serve them steamed or boiled, or add them to dishes such as casseroles and soups. Peas are a good source of protein, carbohydrates, carotenes, B-complex vitamins, vitamin C, vitamin E, copper, iron, phosphorus, and potassium.

Potatoes

These tubers can be used in a multitude of ways—baked, broiled, mashed, and steamed. Use them as the base for other foods such as chili, or add them to soups, casseroles, stews, and salads. Potatoes provide protein, carbohydrates, B-complex vitamins, vitamin C, calcium, iron, and potassium. The peel contains many of the nutrients, so save raw peels for use in making nutritious soup stocks.

Tomatoes

One of the most popular vegetables (technically a fruit), tomatoes are used to make ketchup, pasta sauces, soups, and many other foods. They are available in several different varieties such as Roma, beefsteak, and cherry. Tomatoes are usually eaten when fully ripened, but green tomatoes also can be eaten when thoroughly cooked. Ripe, red tomatoes contain large amounts of vitamin C, especially when raw. Tomatoes also provide carotenes, B-complex vitamins, calcium, magnesium, phosphorus, and potassium.

Sweet Potatoes

Sweet potatoes can be cooked just like regular potatoes, but if anything are even more nutritious. Sweet potatoes contain carbohydrates, fiber, carotenes, vitamin C, calcium, and potassium. The darker the flesh, the more carotenes. They are wonderful when baked and also can be added to baked goods.

Special Note: If your child shows a great dislike for certain fruits, such as grapefruit, and vegetables, such as broccoli, you may have a "taster" on your hands. For many years, it has been known that some people inherit the ability to taste certain bitter substances while others do not. There even appears to be a small percentage of tasters who react even more strongly to these substances—they have been labeled "supertasters."[11] So if your child says a food tastes "yucky" or "bitter," believe it! The solution is not to force your child to eat foods that taste horrible to him or her, but instead to find similar foods that don't contain the offending substances (oranges in place of grapefruits, for example). You also might try cooking the food differently, mixing it with other foods, or adding a small amount of salt to the food as it can block the bitter flavors.

Fruits

Fruits are eaten by just about everyone, no matter what their diet. Fruits are high in carbohydrates, especially sugars, as well as carotenes, vitamin C, calcium, iron, phosphorus, magnesium, chromium, and some B-complex vitamins. They are very low in protein and fat, however, which along with their high sugar content is why they should be eaten in moderation. Dried fruits often contain concentrated quantities of iron and other minerals, especially the darker dried fruits such as dates, raisins, figs, and apricots. They can be prepared for a baby by soaking them in warm water until soft and plump, and then grinding them through a baby food grinder.

Because of their high vitamin C content, fruits have the amazing and important quality of being able to increase the amount of iron that a person can utilize. Orange juice, for example, is an ideal breakfast drink, since the iron in foods like grain cereals and eggs is much more accessible when combined with vitamin C. Lemon juice in water or on a salad, or a fresh fruit dessert, can accomplish the same thing.

The natural sugars in fruit can be easier on the body than

processed sugars because the fiber somewhat slows their digestion and prevents large fluctuations in blood sugar levels. The predominant sugar in fruits, fructose, also is more slowly metabolized than other sugars. Fruits and their juices can be a good source of extra water and quick energy on a hot or exhausting day. More than four ounces a day of fruit juice should not be given to a baby, however, as it can displace other foods. It's also best not to give fruit juice through a bottle, especially at nap or bedtime, as it can contribute to early tooth decay.

Ripe fruits are preferable to green ones because the high starch content of green fruits changes into simple sugars as the fruit ripens, making it easier to digest. For this reason, very ripe bananas are the best first fruit to give to babies, because they are wonderfully digestible in their mushiest state. Avocado, although generally classified as a vegetable, is actually a fruit which happens to be another great choice for a baby food. In addition to being soft and creamy, avocados are unique in being very high in the fats a baby needs.

To obtain the highest quality ripe, unbruised fruits, look for fresh fruit grown locally and in season. In the United States, apples, pears, persimmons, cranberries, and citrus fruits are fall/winter fruits while other berries, melons, peaches, cherries, and plums are spring/summer fruits, although modern supermarkets are fast blurring such distinctions. Bananas are not really a local fruit except in warmer climates, but are available everywhere pretty much all year round. You also will have a choice of other tropical fruits, especially in the summer, such as kiwis, pineapple, papaya, and mango. When a variety of fresh fruit is not available, frozen fruits and juices are the next best thing, and they easily can be added to smoothies or made into sauces for pancakes. If canned fruits are used, choose brands packed in fruit juice or water rather than syrups.

When buying fruit, it is useful to know how picking has affected it. The ideal situation is to have your own fruit trees, and to pick fruit when it is ripe and you are ready to eat it, but this option is seldom practical. Some fruits, such as citrus fruits, melons, peaches, nectarines, berries, and some varieties of apples, do not ripen substantially after picking so if you buy them green, they probably won't ripen enough to feed to your baby. Most other fruits do continue to ripen at room temperature after they have been picked, especially if placed in a bowl with other fruits or in a paper bag. Fully ripened fruit should be stored in the refrigerator or freezer.

As with vegetables, there are so many varieties and types of fruits that only a few of the most popular are discussed below.

Apples

Whether juiced, baked, sauced, dried, or eaten raw, apples are probably the most popular fruit, with thousands of varieties grown throughout the world. Some varieties are better for baking, others for cooking, and yet others for eating raw. In general, apples provide carbohydrates, fiber, carotenes, B-complex vitamins, vitamin C, and traces of several minerals.

Avocados

The rich, green flesh of the avocado is always eaten raw. Spread it on toast, use it in salads, or make it into a guacamole dip. Nutritionally, avocados are a good source of fat as well as providing carbohydrate, protein, fiber, carotenes, B-complex vitamins, vitamin C, calcium, iron, magnesium, phosphorus, and potassium.

Bananas

The first fruit usually given to babies, bananas contain carbohydrates, carotenes, B-complex vitamins, vitamin C, magnesium, potassium, and other minerals. They are usually eaten by themselves but also are wonderful when baked, dried, or added to smoothies, fruit salads, or baked goods.

Berries

The variety of commonly-eaten berries includes strawberries, blackberries, blueberries, cranberries, gooseberries, and raspberries. In general, berries contain carbohydrates, fiber, vitamin C, carotenes, vitamin B-complex, and traces of minerals. Most berries are delicious when eaten raw. Berries also can be made into jams, blended into smoothies, or used in baked goods such as pancakes, muffins, and pies.

Citrus Fruits

The citrus fruits include grapefruits, limes, lemons, mandarin oranges, oranges, pomelos, tangelos, and tangerines. They contain large amounts of vitamin C as well as carotenes, calcium, magnesium, and potassium. The white pith contains bioflavinoids, but most children will refuse to eat it as it is very bitter, although juicing can sometimes disguise the taste. In addition to eating citrus fruits raw or as juice, add them to both vegetable and fruit salads or use them to garnish cooked dishes. Lemon and orange zest (the outer peel, preferably from organically grown fruits) are wonderful in baked goods. Peeled, frozen lemon slices can be used like ice cubes in water or tea.

Figs

Figs are actually a cluster of fruits that appear to be seeds. They may be eaten raw, cooked, or dried. Children especially love them in cookies. Figs contain abundant amounts of carbohydrates, protein, fiber, calcium, iron, magnesium, phosphorus, and potassium. They also provide carotenes and B-complex vitamins as well as a small amount of fat, which is unusual for a fruit.

Melons

From cantaloupe to honeydew to watermelon, these fruits are sure to be a hit with your baby. Melons are eaten raw, either by themselves or in fruit salads, and also are great when juiced. The main nutrient in melons is carbohydrate, but they also can contain significant amounts of carotenes, B-complex vitamins, vitamin C, calcium, phosphorus, and potassium.

Peaches

Along with their relatives, apricots and nectarines, peaches are among the tastiest fruits when picked fully ripe. Eat them as is or use them in salads, smoothies, and baked goods. They also can be dried or sauced. Nutritionally, peaches contain carbo-hydrates, carotenes, and traces of various minerals. When dried, the nutrients are concentrated at which point they become good sources of calcium, iron, magnesium, and potassium.

Eggs

Eggs usually are separated into yolks and whites when feeding them to a baby. The yolk is very high in cholesterol and saturated fat, but nonetheless is an excellent source of protein and fat as well as vitamin A, B vitamins (including vitamin B-12), vitamin D, vitamin E, iron, calcium, zinc, copper, phosphorus, and potassium. The white contains mostly protein. Egg yolk is usually fed to babies before egg white because of the relative indigestibility of the latter. Whole eggs and egg whites should not be given to babies under a year old due to possible allergic reactions. Families with a history of allergies might want to wait until 18 to 24 months. This proscription includes eggs in baked goods, so carefully read the labels of commercial products.

Because eggs can be major carriers of salmonella, *E. coli*, and other potentially dangerous organisms, eggs from factory-farmed hens should be avoided if at all possible. Since essentially all commercial eggs are produced on such farms, this means either keeping your own flock or searching out local eggs from a friend or reputable small farm. But even fresh eggs from free-ranging chickens should be handled as though they are contaminated.

Buy only intact, fresh eggs. Avoid cartons with any sign of broken eggs, feathers, or dung. Do not wash the shells as they are porous and contaminants can be forced inside the egg. Store the eggs in a carton in the refrigerator, separated from other foods, and wash your hands carefully any time you touch them. When using eggs, cook them thoroughly, which means hard-boiling, thorough scrambling, or baking. Never feed your child raw cookie dough, soft-boiled eggs, or other products containing raw or undercooked eggs. After preparing eggs, clean the work area and all utensils thoroughly, and mop up spills with paper towels rather than a sponge. Bacterial contamination can be reduced or eliminated by allowing kitchen surfaces and sponges to dry out thoroughly between uses or by regularly cleaning them with diluted bleach.

Dairy Products

Animal milks are no substitute for breast milk or formula, and cows' milk is the number one cause of allergies in children, so milk and dairy products should not be fed before 12 months. However, since animal milks, and many of the dairy products made from them, contain substantial protein, vitamin A, B vitamins (including vitamin B-12), vitamin K, calcium, and other essential minerals (with the notable exception of iron), you may want them to be a part of your toddler's diet. This is fine so long as dairy products don't supplant other foods, and your child doesn't develop allergies or iron-deficiency anemia, or become lactose-intolerant.

Cows' milk often has supplemental vitamin D added. In addition, whole cows' milk contains ample fat, much of it saturated, and all milk has a small amount of cholesterol. Reduced fat milk contains about half as much fat as whole milk while skim milk contains essentially no fat. Because young children have a greater need for fat, whole-fat dairy products are preferable during the first two years of life.

Although cows' milk is usually what is meant by "milk," lacto-vegetarians can vary their diet by also including products made from the milk of sheep, goats, and other animals. Many people actually prefer products such as goats' milk and sheep cheese. These alternative products usually are less available than cows' milk products, however, and often are more expensive. Also, as mentioned in chapter two, unfortified goats' milk and formula is low in folacin and pyridoxine.

Although raw milk, and the products made from it, supposedly are produced in a cleaner and more natural environment, they should not be fed to young children. Babies are very vulnerable to food poisoning organisms. Even pasteurized products should be handled carefully. Buy milk well before the expiration date, store it in the refrigerator, use it quickly, and throw it out if it develops any odor or shows signs of thickening.

One of the most popular of all dairy products is yogurt, which is made by adding a bacterial culture to warm milk and allowing the bacteria to grow. The bacteria will be killed during pasteurization, but some products have live cultures added which are claimed to aid digestion. Whether it is healthier than other milk products or not, yogurt is delicious and can be a good addition to your toddler's diet. Yogurt can be made from many kinds of animal milk (and non-dairy milks), but yogurt from cows' milk is most common in the United States. For your baby, choose whole-fat, plain yogurt and add fruits and sweeteners at home. You also might try the yogurt-like beverage, kefir.

Soft cheeses like cottage cheese and ricotta, and harder cheeses like Jack and cheddar, are good sources of protein, fat, vitamin A, riboflavin, calcium, phosphorus, and potassium. Because most of the lactose is converted to lactic acid during processing, cheese is more digestible than milk. Soft cheese will be easier for a child to eat. Save the harder cheeses for when your child can chew them properly, or melt them onto toast, pasta, pizza, or vegetables. Finally, remember that almost all aged cheeses are coagulated with animal rennin, an enzyme obtained from the stomachs of veal calves, or pepsin, from sheep and pigs. Look for aged cheeses made with a vegetable rennin, or use only fresh cheeses, which are cultured with lactic acid, lemon juice, or other vegetarian ingredients.

Although butter is made from milk products and contains vitamins A and D, the fat content of this food is quite concentrated and mostly saturated, and so should be used only sparingly, if at all. Foods for young babies should not be fried.

Supplementary Foods

A number of spices, natural food enhancers, and herbs are also good for babies (and for parents). Some of these foods contain concentrated amounts of healthy substances which can enhance a vegetarian diet. Others have useful cooking properties. They can be introduced near the end of the first year as the dishes you feed your baby become more complicated. A few of the most common and popular supplementary foods are described below.

Carob

Although chocolate, which is a processed form of the cocoa bean, is actually a perfectly fine food when eaten in moderation, many people prefer to use carob as it has similar properties while being caffeine-free and much lower in fat. Carob is the seed of the carob tree, and it comes in both powders and syrups. Use carob products as you would similar chocolate products. Be on guard, however, against carob "health food" treats which have large amounts of added hydrogenated fats and sweeteners. Nutritionally, chocolate might be the better choice.

Garlic

You won't want to feed garlic to a baby, but some toddlers and older children love it. The health properties of garlic are too well known to need repeating here. If your child likes it, go ahead and use it in his or her foods as you would any herb.

Nutritional Yeast

Red Star Brand Vegetarian Support Formula nutritional yeast comes either in flaked or powdered form. They are the same— just use twice as much of the flakes as you would the powder in any given recipe. You also can make your own powder from the flakes simply by running them through a small grinder or rubbing them between the palms of your hands. Nutritional yeast can be used rather like Parmesan cheese. Sprinkle it onto pasta, popcorn, or vegetables. It also gives a nice flavor and yellow color to vegan French toast and vegan macaroni & "cheese." Because it is fortified with vitamin B-12, nutritional yeast is highly recommended for use by vegans and near-vegans. For ideas on how to use nutritional yeast, consult *The*

Nutritional Yeast Cookbook: Recipes Using Red Star Vegetarian Support Formula by Joanne Stepaniak (Book Publishing Company, 1997).

Lecithin

Lecithin is a group of substances found in the nerves and blood of animals and the tissues of plants. Since our bodies synthesize it, there appears to be no reason to take it as a supplement, especially since it supplies as many calories as a fat. However, because it is an emulsifier, lecithin can be used as a very effective egg replacer in many baked goods. Some people also like the taste of the granules when sprinkled onto foods or mixed into beverages. Although lecithin is a major ingredient of egg yolk, commercial lecithin generally is derived from soybeans.

Molasses

When sugar cane or sorghum are refined, a thick syrup which contains essentially all the nutrients of the original plant remains. Blackstrap molasses is the most nutrient-dense, and it is an excellent source of iron and calcium. Other types of molasses supply minerals, as well. Use molasses to flavor hot cereal or in baked goods such as gingerbread. Some children like to dip vegetables into it. You also can serve your child a molasses "tea" made by mixing a tablespoon of dark or blackstrap molasses into a cup of hot water. Not every child will like the strong flavor, but if yours does, it makes a healthful treat.

Sea Vegetables

Small amounts of sea vegetables are an excellent way to supply minerals to your child's diet, including iodine, iron, and calcium. Try different ones—dulse, hijiki, Irish moss, kelp, kombu, nori, sea lettuce, sea palm, wakame—to find which your child likes best. Since sea vegetables also contain large amounts of sodium and B-12 analogs, it is best not to overdo them. Serve them at lunch or dinner two or three times a week. A good sea vegetable cookbook is *The Sea Vegetable Gourmet Cookbook and Wildcrafter's Guide* by Eleanor Lewallen and John Lewallen (Mendocino Sea Vegetable Company, 1996).

Processed Foods

A distinction needs to be made between processing and refining. While the latter often strips foods of their nutritive value, the former can make foods more readily accessible and easy to use. Occasionally, processing may even make them more nutritious, as in the case of fortified soy milks or molasses.

In general, look for processed foods made from whole ingredients, preferably organically grown. Add a few low-fiber foods such as pasta made from semolina flour because your child will be able to eat and absorb more calories due to their reduced bulk. Minimal packaging is a plus for the environmentally aware, and lined cans, often used by health food manufacturers, can protect your child from exposure to potentially toxic metals. Use these foods when you don't have the time or the inclination to make things from scratch or when fresh ingredients are not available. Canned beans, frozen fruits and vegetables, tetrapak tofu, bulk pasta, instant oatmeal, dried fruits, and many other processed foods can make all the difference between an interesting, varied, nutritionally sound diet and an overly restrictive one. Use them when you need or want to with a clear conscience.

Feeding Guidelines

A well-selected vegetarian diet is in harmony with the laws of nature and will help assure a healthy, vital, and strong body which serves as the temple for our thoughts, feelings, and spiritual essence.

Nathaniel Altman, from *Eating for Life*[1]

Dietary habits that are well established by age eight to ten will likely last a lifetime.

Charles R. Attwood, M.D.[2]

Birth to Four Months

Overview

BREAST MILK or formula should be your child's basic source of nutrition for the first 12 months. But while you don't have to worry much about his diet, you need to establish a regular pattern of feedings and make sure that he's getting enough calories for growth.[3]

Breast milk is acknowledged to be the ideal food for infants, and, if the mother is eating well and taking care of herself, it will satisfy all a baby's nutritional needs. Unfortunately, less than 60 percent of American women choose to breast-feed, and most of those breast-feed for less than six months, despite the fact that "five to six months postpartum [is] the period of breast-feeding recommended as most critical for the infant's health by the Surgeon General of the United States."[4] By choosing to breast-feed your own child, you not only will be doing what is best for him or her, but you also will be setting a good example for others.

Not everyone is able to breast-feed, despite the best of intentions. Children who are adopted or fostered generally cannot be fed breast milk, and a very small percentage of women experience insurmountable difficulties such as not producing enough milk or not being able to master the skill of nursing. A mother might become so ill that she cannot nurse, and many women have no choice but to return to a workplace that does not accommodate nursing mothers. Breast surgery, which has become more common in recent years both for medical and cosmetic reasons, also can compromise a woman's ability to nurse.

While the ideal is to breast-feed for two or more years, if you only can breast-feed for one year, or six months, or six weeks, or one week, then do so. If you cannot breast-feed at all, or must stop well before your child is ready to be weaned, the next best thing is to feed your baby a high-quality commercial infant formula. Homemade formulas should never be used. (*Note:* Another option is milk from another woman, either directly, in the old-fashioned sense of a wet-nurse, or through a modern milk-bank. Unfortunately, neither option is practical in most cases. However, if you have a plentiful milk supply, you might consider donating milk to others.)

Breast-feeding

There are 4,000 species of mammals, and they all make a different milk. Human milk is made for human infants and it meets all their specific nutrient needs.

Ruth Lawrence, M.D.[5]

Breast-feeding starts before birth. In the past, girls and young women learned to breast-feed by watching their mothers, aunts, sisters, cousins, and friends feeding their own children. Today, with breast-feeding largely relegated to the bedroom or public restroom, and babies carefully tucked underneath the mother's garments when in view of others, few opportunities exist to learn by direct observation. So if you plan to breast-feed, and you have not learned with previous children, you will need to educate yourself thoroughly on the subject before your baby is born. Since this is not a book on breast-feeding, only the most general directions can be given, but the basics are as follows.

1. Begin nursing your baby as soon as possible, preferably within an hour of birth. This first nursing is more of a learning and bonding experience than a serious feeding, but it will set the stage for the future. Newborns have such a powerful instinct to nurse that, when placed on top of their mothers, they can find the breast unassisted within the first hour after birth; later, they lose this ability.

2. Experiment with different positions and possibly props, such as pillows, until you find the most comfortable and effective method for you and your infant.

3. Learn to help your baby latch on to your breast and suck well. A lactation specialist, midwife, or an experienced friend or relative can help with this step. Books and videos also can provide visuals which will aid you in learning the techniques of breast-feeding so you can avoid needless soreness and frustration.

4. Suckle your child as often as you can in order to establish a good milk supply. While you're still in the hospital, do not allow the staff to put you on a rigid nursing schedule, and do everything you can to have your infant in your room with you. Infants can nurse as often as every hour, and most will nurse every two hours or so at the beginning. Schedules which have you nursing every three or four or more hours can interfere with the development of your milk supply while needlessly frustrating your baby. Later, you will establish a reasonable schedule for your child, but at the beginning, let your infant decide what he or she needs.

5. Do not allow others, especially at the hospital, to give your

baby bottles or pacifiers. Later on this isn't so much of a problem, but an infant can become confused by artificial nipples, and feedings of water or formula can interfere with your baby's appetite, resulting in reduced sucking and poor milk production.

6. The first feedings will be of small amounts of colostrum with the milk gradually coming in within a few days of delivery and maturing over the course of the following weeks. The duration of nursing sessions will increase and their frequency decrease as you produce more milk, as the nutritional profile of the milk changes, and your baby matures.

7. Note that Dr. Spock specifically states that "babies normally lose weight in the first few days" after birth. If this happens, recognize it as normal and not a result of inadequate breast-feeding, and be assured that "breast-fed babies will gain the weight back as soon as their mother's milk comes in."[6]

8. Observe your baby while nursing so you can recognize his or her individual nursing pattern. This naturally will change over time, but with careful observation, you will notice any abrupt changes and be able to respond quickly if a problem develops.

9. Be assured that a baby who is allowed to breast-feed on a self-demand schedule, with no impediments, will take in precisely the right amount of milk needed for optimal growth. A baby will nurse more often to increase the milk supply if he or she is still hungry. This is a natural balancing mechanism between the mother and child so that the baby will not go hungry.

10. If your baby seems hungry after nursing, let him or her nurse more often to increase your milk supply. If this procedure does not work, check with your doctor to make sure the child is gaining enough weight, or to find out if there might be some other problem which just seems like hunger.

11. Give your child loving attention at times other than nursing so food is associated more with physical hunger than with love and affection.

12. While the need for a baby to nurse should be respected, limits should be observed as breast-feeding can tax a woman, especially if she is unable to sleep and rest well enough. The mother's main nutritional responsibility toward her child at this time is to take care of herself with rest and a good diet with plentiful calories and fluids. This is especially true if the birth was hard or a Caesarean section was performed.
13. Once breast-feeding and your milk supply are well established, continue until your child naturally weans, your milk supply naturally diminishes, or you want or need to stop nursing.
14. Don't allow anyone to tell you that your shouldn't be breast-feeding or that your child is too old to be nursing. If they do anyway, don't listen!

For more information on breast-feeding, ask your physician or a nurse-practitioner for assistance. As mentioned in chapter three, groups for nursing mothers, such as the International Childbirth Education Association or La Leche League, can be an invaluable resource, as can an experienced midwife. Many of the books mentioned in previous chapters include information on breast-feeding, including those by Dr. Spock and La Leche League. The additional titles listed below also are excellent.

RESOURCES

So that's what they're for!: Breast-feeding Basics by Janet Tamaro (Adams Media Corporation, 1998).

Lactation Specialist Self-Study Series: Modules 1–4 by Rebecca F. Black, Leasa Jarman, and Jan B. Simpson (Jones and Bartlett, 1998). This series of books is written for professionals but is very informative and relatively easy to read. Get them if you want more information than is available in more general books.

Commercial Infant Formulas

If the parents have chosen not to breast-feed or if breast-feeding is discontinued before the baby is year-old, a commercially prepared infant formula should be used. Infant formulas are modeled after breast milk and follow standards set by the Infant Formula Act of 1980, which assure that they contain safe and adequate levels of vitamins and minerals.

The Yale Guide to Children's Nutrition[7]

There will, of course, be times when it is not possible to breast-feed your baby, and once your milk supply is established, you can give your child a bottle as often as once a day without compromising nutrition or lactation.[8] As discussed above, if you must for some reason exclusively bottle-feed instead of breast-feeding, you certainly can do so without harming your baby.

While certainly not the equivalent of mother's milk, commercial formulas do contain adequate nutrition. Such formulas have been carefully designed and are improving all the time as nutrition science increases our knowledge of the composition of human breast milk.[9] Homemade formula, no matter how excellent the ingredients, cannot begin to supply similar nutrition. If you want to feed your child a natural diet, choose breast-feeding; otherwise, use a commercial product.

Many different types and brands of formula are available, and which you choose will depend on availability, cost, quality of ingredients, method of preparation, and ethical beliefs. Be aware that both cows' milk and soy formulas can cause allergies as they both contain foreign proteins which are major allergens for humans. Monitor your baby, and if any signs of allergy or chronic indigestion develop, ask the pediatrician about switching to another formula. Hypoallergenic formulas made from specially processed cows' milk are available for children who are allergic to standard cow- and soy-based formulas.

Vegans with an allergic child who for some reason is not being breast-fed may have to compromise in order to feed their child an adequate diet. Consider that a soy allergy during the first few months of life can result in a child who later is unable to eat the soy foods that are such an important part of most vegan diets. Early allergies to one food also can result in the development of allergies to other foods, such as nuts or glutinous grains. A hypoallergenic dairy-based formula now could mean a lifetime of healthy vegan eating later.

If you are feeding your baby a formula either occasionally or regularly, you will need to be much more aware of how much he or she drinks. The need to suck and the need for nourishment are hard to separate clearly for the bottle-fed baby. While the breast empties quickly and the baby can then suck as long as desired without overeating or taking in too much air, the bottle-fed baby gets a steady stream of milk as long as he or she nurses. If your child is overeating, you might try nipples with finer holes so that the milk comes out more slowly, lengthening the amount of time the baby can suck without taking in too much food. Watch your baby carefully for signs of fullness or gas, and don't press more milk formulas upon him or her in an effort to achieve a daily quota. Babies generally can tell you what they need if you listen. Of course, signals can get mixed, so ask your pediatrician for more specific information if you feel there is a problem.

Four to Nine Months

Because the first solid foods for infants are always cereals, fruits, and vegetables, recommendations for introducing these foods are exactly the same for vegetarian infants as for those in omnivorous households.

Mark and Virginia Messina[10]

Overview

From about four months on, a baby is getting ready to eat solid foods. Fruits, vegetables, and easily digested grains are good foods to offer gradually over the course of these months. The order in which foods are offered should take into account digestibility and likelihood of creating allergy. For this reason, most parents start with iron-fortified infant rice cereal as it is hypoallergenic, easily digestible, and sweet. The added iron is thought to be necessary because a baby's need for iron is on the rise at this time. Millet and quinoa are other non-glutinous grains which can be introduced after your infant is accustomed to rice cereal. Quinoa is especially good for babies as it contains a high level of good quality protein as well as having a naturally high iron content. (*See Grains, page 165, for more details on order of introduction as well as cooking directions.*)

A ripe banana is the first fruit in many cultures. Banana not only is extremely digestible, but sweet, and so is a positive introduction to the world of fruits and vegetables. Avocado, papaya, applesauce, stewed apricot, puréed carrot, and baked or boiled sweet potato are examples of other fruits and vegetables to offer early. Many people choose to start with these foods before introducing grains, and that is perfectly acceptable if you prefer to do it that way.

Although a parent can feed some foods to a baby at about four months, it is not necessary to do so until about six months of age, particularly if the baby is breast-fed or your family has a history of food allergies. Waiting longer than six months is not recommended, however, as your child then could find it more difficult to learn to eat solids and could begin to become malnourished. Give only one new food to your baby every three to five days. If the child is allergic or sensitive to a particular food, you will know immediately which one it is and be able to screen it out until the child is older, preventing a more serious and long-lasting allergy.

Begin by giving the baby a taste of whatever new solid food you are introducing. At first, feed solids once a day an hour or so after a normal breast- or bottle-feeding; later, you can switch the order. A traditional way to prepare foods for babies at this age in many cultures is for the parent to chew the food and then offer it to the child. In this way the food is partially digested by the parent's saliva, making it easier for the baby to digest. But go ahead and use the blender or baby food mill if you prefer.

A rough guideline for offering foods follows, keeping in mind that every child is an individual and may be ready for different foods at different times. Continue to nurse or bottle-feed as usual during this time as your baby will continue to need the special nutrition only available from breast milk or formula.

1. Start by offering an iron-fortified infant rice cereal, mixed with breast milk or formula. One-half to one teaspoon is plenty for a first feeding. When your baby is used to the idea, begin to increase the amount gradually to 2 to 4 tablespoons.
2. Either before or after cereal feeding has been established, feed very mushy ripe banana in the same manner.
3. Once the first cereal and fruit are being eaten regularly with no problem, you can begin to offer other soft fruits, such as avocado or papaya, during the next week or two. Vary your offerings, one day giving banana, the next day the other fruit.
4. If your baby is interested, you might start offering two, or even three, meals a day: banana in the morning and avocado at night, for example; or applesauce for breakfast, banana for lunch, and rice cereal for dinner.
5. The next thing to introduce is some of the sweeter vegetables: carrots, sweet potatoes, beets, squash, peas, and baby lima beans. By this time you probably will be regularly serving the baby two or three meals a day. You can add small amounts of juices such as apple or prune juice for a meal-time drink, but not so much as to interfere with nursing. (Note that beets can turn urine and stools a red which looks like blood, but which is harmless.)
6. Try leafy greens which are good sources of calcium and other nutrients: kale, mustard, collards, broccoli, cauliflower, and dandelion greens. High-oxalate vegetables such as spinach, chard, beet greens, and rhubarb also are nutritious but can wait until a little later. Since greens taste a little too strong for most young babies, try mixing them with grain, juice, or other foods. If they still are refused, don't push the matter.
7. Between seven and nine months, some well-cooked and strained legumes can be added. Start with the more easily digestible legumes such as lentils, split peas, and chickpeas.

When those are established, gradually add beans. Well-cooked soybeans, tofu, and soy yogurt also can be fed at this age, but their introduction should be delayed if your family has a history of allergies. Fortified soymilk also can be introduced, but like juice, it is not a substitute for breast milk or formula. (*See Legumes, page 170, for details on the order of introduction and preparation of legumes.*)

8. During the same time period, lacto-ovo families also can add cottage cheese, cows' milk yogurt, and hard-boiled or scrambled egg yolk. Early introduction of dairy products has been linked to diabetes and allergies, however, so you probably will want to delay all dairy products for at least a full 12 months.

9. Although first feedings will be well-puréed foods fed with a spoon, sometime between seven and nine months your child will begin to be able to handle lumpy foods and finger foods. Miniature frozen bagels are a popular teething food; tofu chunks, shell or macaroni pasta, and other foods which easily dissolve in the mouth also can be offered. As your child becomes adept at chewing, offer harder foods.

10. By nine months of age, your baby can eat almost all foods, with the following exceptions: egg whites, cows' milk, citrus fruits (allergens); nut and seed products (allergens, choking hazard); honey and corn syrup (botulism). Wait until the child is at least one year old before including these items in his or her diet. Other foods to avoid are those that can be a choking hazard, namely hot dogs, whole nuts (especially peanuts), chips, whole grapes, whole berries, dry cereal, chunks of apple, raw carrot, crisp cookies, popcorn, rice cakes, raisins, and hard, round candies. Some of these can be offered after a year if they are cut in such a way that the choking hazard is reduced or eliminated (chop grapes into halves or quarters, for example).

11. Include supplements and fortified foods as necessary, especially vitamin B-12 if your child is vegan or near-vegan.

Self-demand Feeding

If it is assumed that food is readily available and adverse psychological factors are excluded, the infant or child will satisfy energy requirements with precision even though food consumption may be variable at each meal.

Pediatric Nutrition Handbook[11]

Especially as you start, food should not be fed with the intention of assuaging hunger completely, but should rather be seen as a supplement to the milk your baby is getting. Most babies get very excited by these new tastes and will gobble them down as if starving. This can be a sign of strong curiosity and openness as much as of hunger. How much you feed a baby at this age depends entirely on how much he or she will eat. There is no reason to insist that your baby eat a specific amount of food, unless there are complicating circumstances that result in a lack of appetite, weight loss, listlessness, or other signs of illness. In such cases, it is important to be in contact with a doctor to determine why your baby is not eating and to decide on a plan of action. For normal, healthy babies, however, the amount of food eaten is likely to vary from day to day.

This is the basic principle behind the notion of self-demand feeding. If you respect your baby's variable appetite and individual preferences right from the start, your child will be much less likely to develop a psychological problem with food later on.

Babies possess an innate sense of what their bodies need; parents need not worry about their child's diet if a variety of foods is made available, so long as all the nutrients needed for full health and growth are present. Dr. Clara Davis, working at the Children's Memorial Hospital in Chicago during the 1930s, used a diet which attempted to reproduce the diet of "primitive" peoples in her classic experiment on appetite as a guide to children's nutrition. The food list included foods of both animal and vegetable origin, but Dr. Davis stated that the specific foods used were not important, as long as the list adequately provided all the nutrients needed for growth.

Dr. Davis wanted to determine whether or not babies would choose to eat well-balanced meals when given a choice of natural foods. Her study of 15 children, reported in the *Canadian Medical Association Journal* in 1939, supported the hypothesis that babies do have an innate judgment which will keep them healthy. The "trick," however, was to offer only unprocessed, natural foods. The babies, ranging from six to 11 months of age, had never been given any foods to supplement their mothers' breast milk. Each child was offered a tray with a wide variety of foods on it at each meal. Each food was in a separate dish. When a baby reached toward a food, the attending adult would then offer a spoonful of that food. At any point, a baby could refuse or choose any food displayed on the tray. No food was offered without a signal from the baby being fed.

The results of this study were impressive. Although babies went on food "binges" and ate quite unorthodox combinations of foods at various meals, each baby, in his or her own way, ate well-balanced meals, according to nutritional standards. The experiment, which lasted for over a year for most of the babies and up to four years for some of them, produced extremely healthy children. Even the children who drank little milk had excellent bone growth, which undermines the popular idea that bone growth depends upon the substantial calcium intake of milk. Two of the children who displayed signs of rickets at the beginning of the study seemed unconsciously to choose high calcium foods such as cod liver oil in greater quantity, and in effect were able to cure themselves by their diet without any interference from the adults.

Dr. Davis was quick to note that self-selection does not produce healthy babies if the foods are poor in quality. She felt that a parent's responsibility is to offer only nutritionally sound, unprocessed foods of a fairly wide variety. She believed that if children are given natural foods and free choice at each meal, the conflict between appetite and nutritional requirements will be resolved. In reprinting her study, one editor remarked, "children old enough to feed themselves are wise enough to select a balanced diet when given an adequate variety of wholesome foods from which to choose. Their wisdom comes from the appetite, an exquisite mechanism that is foolproof as long as it isn't baffled, misled, or seduced by refined foods . . ."[12]

RESOURCES

Preventing Childhood Eating Problems: A Practical, Positive Approach to Raising Kids Free of Food & Weight Conflicts by Jane R. Hirschmann and Lela Zaphiropoulos (Gurze Designs & Books, 1993).

How to Get Your Kid to Eat . . . But Not Too Much by Ellyn Satter (Bull Publishing, 1987).

Sample Menus

Here are typical month-by-month menus for your baby as he or she begins to eat solid foods. These foods are in addition to breast milk or formula. As the amount of solid food your child eats increases from a teaspoon to several tablespoons to full meals, the amount of breast milk or formula will decrease accordingly. La Leche League suggests gradually reducing the frequency of nursing by omitting "one nursing at a time" while substituting another loving activity so your child won't feel deprived. When your child is comfortable with the new nursing schedule, cut out another time, and so on. How quickly you proceed will depend on your child's reaction as well as how long you wish to nurse, but try to nurse for at least one full year, and preferably two. If that is not possible, you can wean your child onto a formula, and continue feeding that by bottle and cup until final weaning at age two or so.

Five Months

Breakfast: iron-fortified infant rice cereal (nurse as usual)

Six Months

Breakfast: iron-fortified infant rice cereal, banana
Lunch: avocado
Dinner: rice cereal, banana (nurse as usual)

Seven Months

Breakfast: rice cereal, avocado

Lunch: carrots, peas

Dinner: millet, lima beans or kale, apple or pear sauce

Snack: fruit juice (can begin to cut down on nursing over the following weeks, months, or years until your child is fully weaned)

Eight Months

Breakfast: egg yolk or tofu pieces, stewed prunes

Lunch: beets, bread, applesauce

Dinner: barley, lentils, yellow squash

Snacks: avocado, banana, fortified soy milk

Nine Months

Breakfast: oatmeal cooked with soft dates

Lunch: sweet potato, collards, yogurt

Dinner: lentils, rice, applesauce

Snacks: banana, bread

— *or*

Breakfast: rice cereal, apricots, fortified rice milk

Lunch: hummus, dates, carrots

Dinner quinoa, peas, mung beans

Snacks: fruit juice, tofu pieces

— *or*

Breakfast: bulgur, figs

Lunch: cabbage, split-pea soup

Dinner: tofu, broccoli, pear

Snacks: cheese, soft crackers

Nine to Fourteen Months

Overview

By nine months of age, a baby is eating on an adult schedule: three meals a day, plus snacks maybe once or twice a day, depending on hunger levels. Snacks that are nutritious and contain little or no added sugars are very important in the diet of a young baby. There is no need to worry about "spoiling a baby's appetite." If your child eats no junk food, then you do not have to be concerned about her or him getting enough nutrition; just prepare attractive meals and feed your child with love and pleasure.

A general food guide is given below which will meet the nutritional requirements for a baby from 12 to 24 months of age. Starting in the ninth month, begin gradually to increase the amount of food your baby is eating until his or her diet approaches the one outlined below. Don't be bothered if your child refuses to eat the recommended number of foods from every group every day. Everyone goes on "food jags" now and then, especially children as they experiment with their likes and dislikes. As discussed in detail above, if offered a variety of healthy foods, your child most likely will eat a balanced diet over time.

In using the guidelines, remember that a "serving" is defined differently for toddlers than for adults—a serving of oatmeal is a quarter cup for a child instead of the half cup an adult would eat, for example. Serving sizes for children are defined as follows:

Grains

  1/2 slice bread

  1/4 cup cooked grain or
    hot cereal

  1/4 cup cooked pasta

  1/2 cup cold cereal

Vegetables

  1/2 cup salad greens

  1/2 cup raw vegetable pieces

  1/4 cup cooked vegetables

  1/3 cup vegetable juice

Legumes

  1/4 cup cooked legumes

  1 ounce tofu

Fruits

  1/2 large or 1 small whole fruit

  1/3 cup fruit chunks

  1/3 cup fruit juice

Nut and Seed Products

  1/3 cup nut or seed milk

  4 teaspoons nut or seed butter

Dairy Products

  1 ounce hard cheese

  1/4 cup cottage cheese

Eggs

  1 hen's egg

Serving sizes can give you an idea of how much to offer, but when it comes right down to it, there really is no need to measure; each day, just give your child foods from each group, using the following guidelines (adapted from guidelines in the original *Vegetarian Baby* and in *Becoming Vegetarian* by Vesanto Melino, Brenda Davis, and Victoria Harrison) to ensure a good balance of nutrient intake, and allow your child to eat until satisfied. It is a good idea to make one of the grain servings an iron-fortified infant cereal, and one of the vegetable servings a green, leafy vegetable.

Lacto-Ovo Vegetarian Child

Vegetables: 2 to 3 servings
Fruits: 2 to 3 servings
Grains: 2 to 5 servings
Legumes or Egg: 1 to 1 1/2 servings
Nut and Seed Products (after 12 months): 1/2 to 1 serving
Dairy Products: 1 serving plus 20 ounces of breast milk, formula, and/or whole cows' milk

Vegan Child

Vegetables: 2 to 3 servings
Fruits 2 to 3 servings
Grains:: 2 to 5 servings
Legumes: 1 to 2 servings
Nut and Seed Products (after 12 months): 1 to 2 servings
Dairy Products: 20 ounces of breast milk and/or formula
Vitamin B-12 supplement

Meal Examples

Six primary kinds of meals are commonly given to a baby from nine to 14 months old, varying mainly in terms of the kind and extent of preparation needed. As a rule, it is good to have one fairly smooth (blended) dish per meal and at least one food that the baby can feed himself or herself.

Young palates become more sensitive when they are exposed

to a wide variety of foods and textures. Some of the tastiest foods can also be the simplest to prepare so there is no need to spend hours in the kitchen in order to offer your child a variety of interesting items. With a philosophy of simplicity in mind, this section includes a list of quick snacks rather than more involved recipes which require a parent at home with little else to do other than shop and cook.

Multi-Dish Meals

Multi-dish meals are an extension of the single food approach used with younger babies, but a wider variety of foods is offered at each meal. Depending on the foods chosen, multi-dish meals usually can be prepared very quickly. Since this type of meal consists simply of small portions of several kinds of foods that have been mashed or puréed, recipes per se are not included here. The guidelines for a daily diet given in the previous section will give you an idea of sample menus. Also, you can put any single food from your own meal, such as baked sweet potato, through the baby food grinder rather than making a completely separate set of foods.

Blender Meals

Blender meals allow you to make quick, whole foods such as juices, smoothies, nut and seed milks, and some types of soups (both hot and cold). Use a blender, food processor, juicer, or grinder as seems most appropriate. For maximum nutrition, serve raw foods such as juices as soon as possible after they are made. Put the food through a fine mesh strainer before feeding it to a younger child.

Because the availability of fresh fruits and vegetables varies with the season, only general recipe guidelines are given here. Blackstrap molasses, nutritional yeast, and wheat germ can be added for extra nutrition if your child likes them. Tofu, milks, and yogurts can be added to juices for more of a milkshake consistency.

Fruit juices: Almost any fresh fruit can be combined or used alone, with water or a milk to thin it down. Some children enjoy the addition of nutritional yeast, frozen banana, or fruit sorbet.

Vegetable juices: Mix two or more vegetables with a little water until completely blended. You won't need to use water if you use a juicer, but your child might like the juice better if it is diluted. Carrots, celery, tomatoes, beets, spinach, parsley, and watercress are especially good for vegetable juices.

Sprout drinks: Because bean sprouts are so small and require good chewing for proper digestion, blending them with other vegetables or fruits is an excellent way to introduce them to your child.

Mixed fruit and vegetable juices: Some fruits and vegetables can be combined for a surprisingly good taste. Examples include apple juice and carrots, or beets and watermelon.

Soups: Cook several small chunks of one or more vegetables (green beans, squash, carrots, cabbage, potatoes, spinach, broccoli, etc.). When the vegetables get soft, add cow or soy milk to the water so that there is about three times as much liquid as vegetable. Butter, olive oil, or light seasonings also can be added to the liquid. Run the vegetables and broth through the baby food grinder or a blender for a delicious cream of vegetable soup in baby portions. Soups can be served hot or cold (but to neither extreme for a baby). Breads and crackers can be soaked in the soup if the child can't or doesn't want to eat the soup alone.

Nut and seed milks: Start by grinding the nuts or seeds into a fine powder. Put the powder into a blender, and add enough liquid to process. Flavor the milk with sweeteners, vanilla extract, and fresh or dried fruits. (*See Nuts and Seeds, page 176, for more details.*)

Fast-Food Meals

Fast-food meals use recipes that call for pre-ground grains, legumes, and sliced vegetables in various combinations. To prepare, cook all ingredients together until they are soft but not runny. Preparation time is about ten minutes, assuming grains and legumes are already ground to a powdery consistency. If you make a large amount, refrigerate or freeze the extra for quick reheating the next day, but don't save foods for more than two to three days unless the portions are frozen. An ice tray makes a good container for freezing small portions of foods. After the food is frozen, pop the cubes out of the tray and store them in a plastic freezer bag that you have labeled with the recipe name and date. To use, thaw the desired amount in the refrigerator, and then reheat.

The recipes in this section are sorted into "breakfast, lunch and dinner" segments, but this is merely tradition, and there is no need to stick to such rigid concepts. If you want to feed your child cereal for dinner, go ahead! Experiment with your own combinations, too.

Breakfast

A combination of grains and fruits, plus chopped nuts for older children, makes a tasty hot cereal that is perfect for breakfast. By using many different ingredients, you can come up with a multitude of dishes which are sure to appeal to a child who has never had standard, processed cereals. Notice that general guidelines are given for making cereals followed by a list of possible combinations, since all of these dishes are prepared in the same manner.

Hot Cereal

   1 tablespoon finely ground whole grain (should be a rough powdery consistency)
   2 pieces dried fruits, pitted and chopped into quarters or even finer
   5 tablespoons milk of your choice

Mix ingredients together, preferably in a small iron pot or skillet. Cook at medium heat for three to five minutes, or until grain and fruit are soft. Add more liquid if necessary to prevent scorching. When the consistency is a solid mush, put the food through a blender or a baby food grinder to further mash the fruit and to thoroughly mix all the ingredients. Cool before serving. (Setting the dish in the freezer for a minute will usually reduce the temperature sufficiently.)

Variations: More than one kind of grain can be used, as well as more than one kind of fruit. Add three tablespoons of liquid for each additional tablespoon of dried grain powder that you add, and two tablespoons for each additional piece of dried fruit. The general cereal recipe provides the approximate amount a child between the ages of ten and sixteen months will eat in one meal. Since appetites vary, you may want to make more or less. If you make too much, you can always cover it tightly and heat it up the next day or serve it cold if your baby likes cool or room-temperature food. A variation is to mix cow or soy yogurt with the cereal to make a smoother, creamier consistency.

Brown Rice Cereal #1: brown rice, pitted dates, almond milk

Brown Rice Cereal #2: brown rice, dried apples or peaches, coconut milk

Barley Cereal: barley, raisins (about seven), cashew milk

Millet Cereal: millet, prunes, coconut milk

Oat Cereal: rolled oats (not instant), apricots, amazake milk

Quinoa Cereal: quinoa, pitted dates, rice milk

Wheat Cereal: wheat flakes, dried figs, ground sesame seeds (about 1/2 tablespoon plus 2 tablespoons extra liquid)

Lunch

For purposes of this section, "lunch" is taken to mean the light meal of the day. This can be noontime, especially when the weather is hot, or evening, if the noon meal is substantial. Timing depends on when your child seems hungriest. In some cultures, the morning meal is the largest one of the day. Whatever time of day you choose, here are some suggestions for combinations of foods. Notice that these meal are largely made from raw foods, which contributes to their light character.

These recipes are all prepared in the same way: simply put all ingredients through a baby food grinder. Nutritional yeast, tahini, blackstrap molasses, wheat germ, and cow or soy yogurt can be added to any of these recipes. As discussed in chapter five, tofu should be rinsed, and possibly steamed, to remove surface bacteria before it is used in a dish that will not be cooked.

Tofu-Raisin Lunch: 1-inch square tofu, 8 to 10 presoaked raisins (soak raisins overnight in small amount of water), 2 tablespoons grated steamed broccoli

Tofu-Banana Lunch: 1-inch square tofu, 1/2 ripe banana, 1/2 tablespoon wheat germ

Tofu-Molasses Lunch: 1-inch square tofu, 1/4 cup fresh lima beans, 1 teaspoon blackstrap molasses

Veggie Lunch: 1/4 steamed zucchini, diced; 1 tablespoon legume sprouts; 1/4 cored, peeled pear

Peas and Tahini Lunch: 1/4 cup green peas; 1/2 cored, peeled apple; 1/2 teaspoon tahini

Fruit and Spouts Lunch: 1 cored, peeled pear; 1 tablespoon legume sprouts; 1 teaspoon nutritional yeast

Walnut Lunch: 1/2 ripe banana; 5 walnuts, finely ground; 1 teaspoon nutritional yeast

Carrot-Yogurt Lunch: 1/2 carrot, grated finely; 8 to 10 presoaked raisins; 2 tablespoons dairy or soy yogurt

Broccoli-Yogurt Lunch: 3 presoaked apricots; 2 tablespoons grated, steamed broccoli; 4 tablespoons dairy or soy yogurt

Cottage Cheese-Apple Lunch: 3 tablespoons cottage cheese; 4 pieces grated apple; 1 tablespoon wheat germ

Cottage Cheese-Nut Butter Lunch: 3 tablespoons cottage cheese, 1 tablespoon smooth nut or seed butter, 2 tablespoons applesauce 1/2 ripe banana

Dinner

Grains, legumes, seeds, and vegetables are used in these heavier "dinner" recipes. All ingredients must be pre-ground, or in the case of vegetables, finely chopped or grated so that they cook as fast as possible, thus reducing any substantial loss of nutrients. If the vegetables are finely chopped, cooking time will be about five to seven minutes at medium heat. After the ingredients are cooked, run them through a baby food grinder to mix them well and improve their texture. Cook ingredients together with the following amounts of water:

3 tablespoons water for each tablespoon ground grain
   or legume
2 tablespoons water for each tablespoon grated vegetable

Barley and Beans Dinner: 1 tablespoon barley; 6 baby lima beans; 1/2 stalk celery, finely sliced; 2 sprigs parsley

Barley and Sweet Potato Dinner: 1 tablespoon barley; 2 1-inch squares sweet potato, finely sliced; 1 tablespoon fresh peas

Buckwheat Dinner: 1 teaspoon buckwheat; 3 medium green beans, finely chopped; 2 apricots

Bulgar Dinner: 1 tablespoon finely ground bulgur; 1/2 tablespoon pinto beans; 1/4 medium beet, finely chopped; 1/4 teaspoon blackstrap molasses

Mexican Dinner: 2 teaspoons brown rice; 1 teaspoon black beans; 1/4 medium summer squash, finely sliced (Cover cooked mixture with melted cheese to make this a good finger food.)

Millet and Green Beans Dinner: 1 tablespoon millet; 1/2 to 1 tablespoon very finely chopped beet greens; 1 tablespoon chopped, steamed cabbage; 1/2 graham cracker or 1/2 tablespoon flour

Millet and Carrot Dinner: 1 tablespoon millet; 1/4 carrot, finely grated; 7 to 8 baby lima beans (A little yogurt added to this mixture after it is cooked makes it smoother.)

Oats and Asperagus Dinner: 1 tablespoons raw, rolled oats; 1 stalk asparagus, finely chopped; 1 tablespoon nutritional yeast, added after other ingredients are cooked; 1/4 cup cow or soy yogurt, added after other ingredients are cooked

Rice and Veggies Dinner: 1 tablespoon brown rice; 1 tablespoon finely grated or sliced broccoli; 1 tablespoon finely sliced summer squash; 1/2 to 1 teaspoon tahini

Rice and Winter Squash Dinner: 1 tablespoon brown rice; 1 tablespoon finely sliced acorn squash; 1 teaspoon nutritional yeast

Rice and Lentils Dinner: 2 tablespoons brown rice; 1 tablespoon lentils; 1 small zucchini squash, finely chopped

Rice and Soybeans Dinner: 1 tablespoon soybeans (preferably precooked or very finely ground into smooth powder); 1 tablespoon brown rice; 1/4 medium tomato, finely blended

Rice and Sprouts Dinner: 1 tablespoon brown rice; 1 tablespoon mung bean sprouts; 3 medium green beans, finely grated or chopped

Spinach Omlette Dinner: 1 egg, scrambled with 1/4 cup milk; 1/2 tablespoon finely chopped spinach (Sauté together in vegetable oil or butter for special taste treat.)

Convenience Meals

Convenience meals have become the choice of many in our fast-paced world. While most convenience foods should be avoided by the health-conscious, food manufacturers have responded to the demand for pre-packaged foods made from whole ingredients, and every day more and more good vegetarian convenience foods enter the market. These include items such as organic vegetarian baby food in jars, whole grain instant infant cereals in boxes, frozen whole grain waffles, mixed frozen fruits for smoothies, exotic nut and seed butters, and brown-rice pudding mixes. Use them when you don't have the time to start from scratch and the alternative is between a whole foods convenience meal and a poor quality junk-food one. Depending upon where you live, you also might be able to find fast-food and family-style restaurants which offer suitable vegetarian dishes made from whole foods.

Adult Adaptation Meals

Adult adaptation meals are exactly what they sound like—dishes taken directly from those which you are eating yourself. The only time to hesitate is when your foods are highly spiced or contain ingredients your baby is still too young to eat. If it won't ruin the dish, you can cook appropriate foods with little or no spice, and then remove a portion for your baby before adding the seasonings. At first, you will need to use a baby food grinder on your child's portion to make a smoother consistency, but as your baby becomes more adept, you can allow him or her to eat small chunks of your meal.

Any vegetarian casserole or main meal for adults can be ground up for a young baby. To provide your family with many nutritious and tasty meals, you will want to look into the enormous number of vegetarian cookbooks that are on the market today. Choose those that contain time-saving recipes, unless you are interested in gourmet cooking. A list of popular books is available at the end of this chapter.

Snacks

In-between meals are often a child's favorite. Make snacks special by arranging a variety of items on a small plate and serving them with a few ounces of fresh juice, smoothie, or your choice of milk. A nice, loving touch is to have your child pick out his or her very own plate, cup, and napkin set to be used exclusively for this purpose.

Ideas for snack foods are given below. Offer only those foods which are age-appropriate, in amounts suited to your child's appetite, and prepare them in a manner your child can safely eat. Experiment with different fruits, vegetables, grain products, protein-fat foods, and beverages until you find the combinations your child likes best. Young children can be overwhelmed by too much choice, so choose a maximum of one item from each of the groups. By preparing foods such as potatoes ahead of time, you can put together a small plate in just a minute or two. Many of these foods also can be offered alone at times when your child needs a small "pick-me-up" and a larger meal is inappropriate, or if you are rushed for time.

Snacks

One-half medium fruit, or equivalent amount of smaller fruits or sauce, prepared as follows:

Apple—peel, if necessary, then cut into narrow wedges

Banana—cut into slices or chunks

Orange or tangerine—remove skin and divide into
sections (cut them in half if necessary)

Seedless grapes—remove from stem and cut in half

Melon—cut into chunks

Strawberries—remove tops and core, then cut into slices
or chunks

Other berries—cut in half

Kiwi—remove skin, then cut into slices or chunks

Dried fruit (except raisins)—cut into pieces, pre-soak
if necessary

Several sticks or small chunks cut from a selection of the following vegetables (steam or blanch hard vegetables for very young children):

Carrot, peeled

Celery, de-"stringed"

Cucumber, peeled

Green peas

Jicama, peeled

Bell pepper, green, red, yellow, orange

Water chestnuts, peeled

Snow peas, blanched or raw

Zucchini, blanched or raw

Broccoli stems and florets, peeled and blanched

Cauliflower florets, blanched

Potato, sweet potato, or beet, cooked and peeled

Two tablespoons of one of the following:

Cooked beans

Hummus

Soft cheese or tofu

Hard dairy or non-dairy cheese, small chunks or melt
onto other food for younger child
Hard-boiled egg yolk (yolk only for child under one year)
Pitted olives, cut in small pieces
Guacamole or avocado, small chunks
Nut or seed butter, smooth

One of the following:

Soft crackers

Pita pocket, 1/2 to 1 small

Corn or flour tortilla, 1/2 to 1 small

Bread, several pieces

Soft granola, small cup

Cold pancake or waffle, half or whole

Fourteen to Twenty-four Months

During toddlerhood the rapid growth of infancy slows and the child's appetite decreases. Often toddlers would much rather play than eat.

The Yale Guide to Children's Nutrition[13]

Overview

By 12 to 14 months of age babies are beginning to feed themselves and can pretty much eat whatever you are eating as long as your foods are not too hot or too highly spiced or filled with inappropriate ingredients such as hard nuts. The pace at which your baby switches to adult-style fare over the course of the second year depends on the child's interest and number of teeth. Without several upper and lower teeth, a baby will still need to have food finely chopped or ground in the baby food grinder, but as your child becomes more adept at chewing, you can feed more and more unprocessed foods.

Remember that children of this age often become picky about their food. Not only does the appetite decrease, but a toddler is so busy exploring that food becomes of secondary interest.

Continue to offer your child a reasonable variety of foods over the course of the day, and try not to become too frustrated when your child refuses the very food that was a favorite the day before. Children of this age especially benefit from a regular feeding schedule with attention paid to mealtime rituals, so do your best to adjust your family schedule appropriately.

The following recipes are sure to be enjoyed by adults as well as children, so adult serving sizes are given. For more ideas, refer to the cookbooks listed at the end of the chapter. By now, what you are eating should be healthy enough that you will not have to think about what to feed your toddler, but if you want more guidance as your child enters the pre-school years, refer to the following books.

RESOURCES

Vegetarian Children by Sharon K. Yntema (McBooks Press, 1995).
Dr. Attwood's Low-Fat Prescription For Kids by Charles Attwood, M.D. (Viking, 1995).

Recipes

Berry Cold & Creamy Smoothie
Amount: 2 to 4 servings (24 to 32 ounces)

2 tablespoons walnut pieces
1 to 2 cups chilled non-dairy or dairy milk
1 package (12.3 ounces) Mori-Nu silken tofu, chilled
1 peeled, frozen banana, cut into chunks
1/2 to 1 cup assorted frozen berries (strawberry, raspberry, blueberry)
1 to 2 tablespoons sweetener
1/2 to 1 teaspoon vanilla extract
Crushed ice (optional)

Place the walnut pieces in a blender and pulse several times to form a grainy powder. Add 1 cup of the milk, and thoroughly blend. Add the tofu, fruit, 1 tablespoon of sweetener, and 1/2 teaspoon of extract, blending until very smooth. Use additional milk as needed, and adjust sweetener and extract to taste. Blend in crushed ice, if desired. Pour into glasses and serve immediately. You may need to make separate batches depending on the size of your blender. You also will want to strain the mixture before serving it to a young child.

Variation: Use chilled pears, melon, or other fruits in place of the berries.

(*Note on sweeteners:* Good granulated sweeteners are Florida Crystals sugar and date sugar. Good liquid sweeteners are maple syrup, barley malt syrup, rice syrup, and liquid Fruit Source. Honey and corn syrup should not be given to a child under a year old.)

Say Sesame Milk

Amount: 1 serving

1 mug-full non-dairy or dairy milk
1/2 tablespoon sesame butter
1 tablespoon sugar

In a small saucepan, heat the milk just to simmering, being careful not to scorch. Remove from heat, add the remaining ingredients, and stir until well mixed. Serve immediately.

Molasses Tea

Amount: 1 serving

1 mug-full boiling water
1 tablespoon blackstrap molasses

Stir the molasses into the hot water until thoroughly dissolved. Serve immediately.

Better Spread

1/4 cup butter   1/4 cup flax seed oil

Pour the flax oil into softened butter and stir until thoroughly mixed. Chill to harden. (Vegans can either substitute margarine for the butter or purchase a similar commercial product which is free of trans-fatty acids: Spectrum Naturals Essential Omega Spread.)

Good Morning Pancakes

Amount: 18 to 24 pancakes

2 1/4 cups whole wheat pastry flour
1 tablespoon baking powder
1/4 to 1/2 teaspoon salt
2 tablespoons granulated sweetener
1/2 teaspoon ground cinnamon
4 1/2 teaspoons Ener-G Egg Replacer powder
6 tablespoons water, non-dairy milk, or dairy milk
2 cups non-dairy or dairy milk
1 tablespoon liquid soy lecithin
1 tablespoon canola oil
Toppings: maple syrup, jam, applesauce, sliced fruits

In a large mixing bowl, sift the flour with the baking powder, salt, granulated sweetener, and cinnamon. Set aside. In a medium mixing bowl, beat the Ener-G Egg Replacer powder with 6 tablespoons of water or milk until frothy. Add the rest of the wet ingredients to the egg replacer mixture and continue to beat until thoroughly combined. Pour the wet mixture onto the top of the dry ingredients, and stir until a slightly lumpy batter forms. Add more flour or milk as needed to adjust the consistency of the batter. For each cake, pour 1/4 cup of batter onto a lightly oiled, hot griddle. Flip with a sharp spatula when bubbles are well formed and the cake is just beginning to look dry around the edge. Brown the other side, and serve immediately with desired toppings. Pancakes also can be frozen and re-heated.

Variations: 1) For waffles, reduce milk to 1-3/4 cups and increase both the soy lecithin and the oil to 2 tablespoons each. 2) Add 1/4 cup of chopped nuts, or fresh or defrosted berries, to the batter. 3) Substitute 1/4 to 1/2 cup of other whole grain flours for the wheat flour. Buckwheat, teff, and cornmeal are especially good.

Rise and Shine Quinoa Cereal
Amount: 1 to 2 servings

1 cup, uncooked, quinoa
2 cups filtered water
1 apple, cubed
1 to 2 tablespoons seeds or chopped nuts
maple syrup
non-dairy or dairy milk

In a fine-mesh strainer, soak and thoroughly rinse the quinoa in cold water to remove the bitter saponin coating. Water should run clear. Place the quinoa and filtered water into a medium-size saucepan. Bring to a boil, reduce to a simmer, cover, and cook for 10 to 15 minutes, until all the water is absorbed. Remove from heat and let sit, covered, for 5 minutes. Fluff with a fork, and place in serving bowls. Add cubed apple, seeds or chopped nuts, maple syrup, and milk to taste. Serve immediately. Peel the apple and omit the seeds or nuts when serving to a young child.

AM/PM Tofu Scramble
Amount: 2 to 4 servings

8 ounces firm tofu, well-drained and patted dry
4 teaspoons nutritional yeast powder
2 teaspoons tamari soy sauce
1/8 teaspoon turmeric
1 tablespoon olive oil
1 small yellow onion, chopped
2 small cloves garlic, minced
1 tomato, coarsely chopped
1 1/2 cups, loosely packed, spinach or Swiss chard leaves

In a large bowl, break up the tofu into small chunks with a fork or your hands. Add the yeast, soy sauce, and turmeric. Gently mix, being careful not to over-mix. The consistency should be similar to scrambled eggs. In a large skillet, heat the oil. Sauté the garlic and onion until softened. Add the tofu mixture along with the tomato and greens. Gently stir until the ingredients are just mixed, then cover for one to two minutes until the greens are wilted. Serve immediately.

Good with whole grain toast, pancakes, or potatoes. Leftovers can be refrigerated and then re-heated or used as a sandwich filling. Since young children often dislike "mixed-up" foods, they might prefer this dish without the vegetables.

Bonzo Spread (hummus)

Amount: 1-1/2 cups

1 to 2 cloves garlic
15 ounces can (about 2 cups) unsalted garbanzo beans (chickpeas)
3 tablespoons tahini
2 tablespoons cold water
4 tablespoons fresh lemon juice
2 tablespoons olive oil
1/2 teaspoon ground cumin
1/2 teaspoon ground coriander
1/2 teaspoon salt
1/4 teaspoon paprika

Rinse and drain the garbanzo beans. In a food processor, mince the garlic. Add all other ingredients except 1 tablespoon of olive oil and the paprika, and process until very smooth, adding more water if necessary. Spread into a shallow 6-inch wide bowl, and sprinkle the surface with the remaining 1 tablespoon olive oil and the paprika. Chill for several hours. Use as a spread for toast or sandwiches, a stuffing for celery logs, a dip for vegetables, or a filling for lightly fried corn or flour tortillas. Children may prefer a less spicy version of this dish.

Macaroni and Cheese

Amount: 4 servings

16 ounces macaroni
8 to 16 ounces orange soy or cows' cheese, grated
1/4 to 1/2 cup soy or cows' milk
2 to 3 teaspoons canola oil (optional)
1/2 teaspoon onion powder
1/2 teaspoon dry mustard
2 teaspoons nutritional yeast powder

Boil macaroni until *al dente.* Drain, place in a large bowl, and set aside. In a saucepan, melt the cheese with the milk. If using soy cheese, add oil as needed to improve the texture. Stir in onion powder, dry mustard, and nutritional yeast powder. When cheese sauce is thoroughly melted, pour over the macaroni, and stir to coat. *Note:* Only non-vegan soy cheese with casein will work satisfactorily in this recipe.

Nut Butter Wrap

1 small flour tortilla
1 to 2 tablespoons smooth nut or seed butter
1 to 2 leaves romaine or green leaf lettuce, whole or
   shredded

Spread the nut or seed butter on the tortilla, and cover with the lettuce. Fold one end of the tortilla over, turn one-quarter turn, and roll the sides to form a tube. Serve. Excellent with Molasses Tea!

Tooty-Fruity Salad

Amount: 4 servings

1 cup apple chunks
1/2 cup pineapple chunks
1/2 cup seedless grapes, halved
2 to 3 ounces fresh orange juice
1 banana, sliced
2 to 4 tablespoons raisins

Place all the fresh fruit and raisins into a bowl. (Peel apples and omit raisins if serving to young children.) Pour the orange juice, 1 tablespoon at a time, over the fruit, using enough juice to coat but not so much that the fruit becomes soggy. Chill in the refrigerator for 1 to 2 hours. *Note:* Can serve immediately if fruit is refrigerated before assembly.

Nut-Yeast Not-Fries
Amount: 2 to 4 servings

2 large russet potatoes, well scrubbed
1 tablespoon olive oil (or olive oil spray)
4 tablespoons nutritional yeast powder
1/4 teaspoon salt
1/8 teaspoon cayenne pepper (optional)

In a large pot, boil the whole potatoes for 25 to 30 minutes until cooked but still firm. Drain the potatoes and plunge them into cool water to reduce their heat quickly. When cool, use a sharp knife to slice the potatoes into strips or rounds, handling carefully to reduce crumbling. Peel if preparing them for young children. Place olive oil in a small, shallow bowl (omit this step if using a spray). In another small, shallow bowl, mix the nutritional yeast powder with the salt and cayenne pepper, if desired. Dip each potato slice or round into the oil (or coat with spray) and then roll in the yeast mixture until well coated. Place the potato pieces onto a lightly oiled or non-stick cookie sheet, and bake at 425° for 5 to 10 minutes until potatoes are golden brown. Serve immediately, plain or with ketchup.

Sweet Orange Sweet Potatoes
Amount: 2 to 3 cups

2 medium-large sweet potatoes
2 to 4 tablespoons fresh orange juice
1 to 2 tablespoons maple syrup
1/4 teaspoon salt
1/2 to 1 tablespoon butter or Spectrum Naturals® spread

Cook the sweet potatoes by any method (bake, boil, micro-wave), and remove the skins. Place the cooked sweet potato flesh into a food processor with the other ingredients. Process until very smooth, adjusting orange juice, syrup, salt, and butter or spread to taste. Spoon mixture into a bowl, and serve. May also be refrigerated for up to several days and either served cold or reheated in a small saucepan or microwave.

English Muffin Pizzaz!

> 2 halves English muffin
> 2 to 4 tablespoons tomato paste or thick red pasta sauce
> 2 slices non-dairy or dairy cheese

Toast the English muffin halves. Spread the tomato paste or pasta sauce onto the faces, place the cheese on top, and broil until the cheese is melted. Let cool slightly, and serve.

Bella's Orange Date Nut Bread
> This recipe courtesy of Sara, lacto-vegetarian mother of near-vegan baby Isabella.
> *Amount:* 1 large loaf

> 3 cups whole wheat pastry flour
> 3 1/2 teaspoons baking powder
> 1 1/2 teaspoons salt
> 2 tablespoons ground flax seeds
> 4 tablespoons water
> 1/3 cup liquid sweetener such as brown rice syrup
>   or honey
> 2 tablespoons canola oil, Spectrum Naturals® spread,
>   or soft butter
> 1 teaspoon vanilla extract
> 1/2 cup fresh orange juice
> Zest from one organic orange
> 1 cup soy or cows' milk
> 1 cup sliced, pitted dates
> 1/2 cup chopped nuts or seeds

In a large bowl, sift together the flour, baking powder, and salt. Set aside. In another bowl, whisk together the ground flax seeds and water. Add the sweetener, oil or butter, vanilla, orange juice, orange zest, and milk to the flax mixture, and stir to blend. Pour the wet mixture onto the dry mixture and stir until just blended. Add the dates and nuts or seeds. Transfer batter to a large greased loaf pan (approximately 9" x 5" x 3"), and bake at 350° for approximately 65 minutes. Cool on rack and remove from pan.

Nut Balls

1/2 cup each:
nut butter
sweet cocoa or carob powder
wheat germ
barley malt syrup
instant cows' or soy milk powder (optional)

Mix together, divide into small lumps or balls, and refrigerate for several hours or overnight.

Rice Pudding

Amount: 4 to 6 servings

2 cups, cooked, basmati or Arborio rice
3 cups non-dairy or dairy milk
1/4 to 1/2 cup sweetener
1/4 to 1/2 teaspoon ground cinnamon or coriander
1/4 teaspoon salt
1 teaspoon vanilla extract
2 to 4 tablespoons, coarsely chopped, almonds or pistachio
nuts (optional)

In a large saucepan, combine all ingredients except the nuts. Bring to a boil, reduce heat, and simmer for 25 to 30 minutes, stirring frequently. Remove from heat, and stir in the nuts, if desired. Spoon into pudding cups. May be served warm or cold.

Note: Coconut milk is especially good in this recipe, but because it is very high in saturated fat it should be reserved for special occasions. You can dilute coconut milk with other milks to have the flavor with less saturated fat. You also can add a small amount of shredded coconut.

Popsicles

Pour any fresh fruit juice other than pineapple into small paper cups or special freezer molds. Insert popsicle sticks or the handles which come with the mold. Freeze until juice is solid. Remove cup by holding stick and running under hot water for about ten seconds. A great variation is to blend a plain yogurt with the fruit juice before freezing the mixture as described.

RESOURCES

Cookbooks Specifically for Children and Families

Better Than Peanut Butter & Jelly: Quick Vegetarian Meals Your Kids Will Love! by Wendy Muldawer and Marty Mattare (McBooks Press, 1997).

Burgers 'N Fries 'N Cinnamon Buns: Low-Fat, Meatless Versions of Fast Foods Favorites by Bobbie E. Hinman (Book Publishing Company, 1993).

From Animal Crackers to Wild West Beans: Easy and Fun Vegetarian Recipes for Healthy Babies and Children by Carol Timperley (NTC/Contemporary Publishing, 1998).

Feeding the Healthy Vegetarian Family by Ken Haedrich (Bantam Doubleday Dell, 1998).

Feeding the Whole Family: Whole-foods Recipes for Babies, Young Children and Their Parents by Cynthia Lair (Moon Smile Press, 1997). This book is not completely vegetarian, but it's very close.

The Vegetarian Lunchbasket: 225 Easy, Nutritious Recipes for the Quality-Conscious Family on the Go by Linda, Haynes (New World Library, 1993).

Vegan Handbook: Over 200 Delicious Recipes, Meal Plans, and Vegetarian Resources for All Ages edited by Debra Wasserman and Reed Mangels (Vegetarian Resource Group, 1996).

Cookbooks with Recipes Suitable for Children

Not Milk . . . Nut Milks: 40 of the Most Original Dairy-Free Recipes Ever by Candia Lea Cole (Woodbridge Press, 1997).

The Uncheese Cookbook: Creating Amazing Dairy-Free Cheese Substitutes and Classic 'Uncheese' Dishes by Joanne Stepaniak (Book Publishing Company, 1994).

Vegan Vittles: Recipes Inspired by the Critters of Farm Sanctuary by Joanne Stepaniak (Book Publishing Company, 1996).

Vegetarian Times Complete Cookbook by the editors of *Vegetarian Times* Magazine (MacMillan, 1995).

The Cookbook for People Who Love Animals by Michael A. Klaper, MD (Gentle World, 1990).

Sweet Temptations Natural Dessert Book by Frances Kendall (Avery Publishing Group, 1988).

Uprisings: The Whole Grain Bakers' Book (Book Publishing Company, 1991).

Luscious Low-Fat Desserts by Marie Oser (Chariot Publishing, 1994).

SEVEN

Questions and Answers

WHILE THE preceding chapters have covered as much ground as possible on the subject of how to feed your vegetarian baby, you still may be left with unanswered questions. This chapter, therefore, includes direct questions asked of the authors during interviews and private conversations. If your concern was not addressed in the preceding text, perhaps you will find an answer here. Where appropriate, references to relevant portions of the text are made so you can go back to look for more information.

If you still have questions concerning your vegetarian baby's diet after reading this chapter, the authors invite you to send queries in care of the publisher. Sharing of information is one of the best ways for us all to learn. Contact the authors:

c/o McBooks Press
120 West State Street
Ithaca, NY 14850
http://www.mcbooks.com; mcbooks@mcbooks.com

Q. How can you raise your children as vegetarians if they don't like vegetables? I thought children usually don't like vegetables, especially when they're young.

A. The concept of a "vegetable war" is a common one among meat-eaters. In fact, there was an article in the September 1978 issue of *American Baby* magazine entitled: "Kids vs. Vegetables: How to Win the War." The stereotype of children hating vegetables is a result of a combination of factors. First, many parents do not like vegetables very much and convey this message to their children even as they are trying to force vegetables on them "because it's good for them." Second, many meat-eaters prepare vegetables only as a side dish and usually do not put the same attention into making them taste good that a vegetarian would. No one likes overdone, soggy vegetables—which also, by the way, have lost a good deal of their nutrients through overcooking.

A third factor is the greater society which, through language, advertisements, and the like, denigrates vegetables and makes it seem that the only way they can be made edible is to slather them with melted cheese and salt or to them in oil. This will be more of a factor with an older child than an infant, but it's amazing what information and attitudes young children pick up through their own observations. You can counteract these societal messages somewhat with pro-vegetable activities like gardening, vegetable-based food play, vegetable coloring books and calendars, vegetable plush toys, and the like.

Finally, as was discussed in chapter five, the lack of interesting varieties of produce grown in season and picked when ripe has resulted in vegetables that—all too often—neither look nor taste particularly good. And remember that there is a possibility that your child is a "super-taster," which can make certain vegetables taste horribly bitter.

So, what's the solution? For the most part, if you give your child food you enjoy—fresh vegetables, not overcooked, at times lightly seasoned or mixed with other favored foods like pasta sauce, yogurt, or nutritional yeast—the "vegetable wars" are much less likely to occur. War exists only if someone is fighting. If parents don't force their children to eat vegetables, sooner or later the children will enjoy eating most vegetables. If you find that hard to believe, go back to chapter three and reread some of the interviews. Several parents emphasized their children's love of a variety of vegetables, so it is definitely possible!

Q. What do I do if my child refuses to eat the foods I prepare? How do I make sure he or she eats enough to get the recommended amounts of all vitamins and minerals?

A. The first thing to do is to figure out why your child isn't eating. There are a number of possible reasons:

1. Your child is sick, in which case you should respect her or his feelings about how much food to eat. You might try offering more soupy or light foods rather than concentrating on a normal meal. Monitor a sick child carefully, however, and contact a doctor if your child's appetite doesn't return within a reasonable amount of time.

2. Your child may not be enjoying mealtimes. Is the eating atmosphere calm and happy? Are you as a parent enjoying these times?

3. Your child is upset about something which has nothing to do with mealtimes or food, but which is interfering with his or her ability to concentrate on or enjoy eating. Life can be very difficult for toddlers, but communication is hard for them, so if your child appears depressed or upset, try to find out why.

4. Your child is becoming more of an individual person. Experimenting with likes and dislikes of certain foods may be part of this development. Such experimentation usually happens during the second year of life, and it is helpful not to make a fuss over it. Serve more of a variety to replace something the child is temporarily refusing to eat, and make sure you are not serving empty-calorie foods, too much juice, or other foods that can take away a child's appetite. Snacks are useful, especially if the child is not eating large amounts at meals, but make sure those snacks are very nutritious. An alternative to offering snacks to the child who is not eating well is to offer only two or three meals a day, and at those meals, to serve nutritious snack-type foods that contain a good balance of essential nutrients. Chapter six offers many suggestions for such foods.

If your child is offered nothing but tasty, nutritious foods, there generally is no need to worry when a period of food refusal or a preference for certain foods comes along unless it goes on for so long that it noticeably begins to affect your child's health. Reread the section in chapter six on self-demand feeding, and consider giving your child an appropriate multi-vitamin/mineral for peace of mind. Also keep in mind the following wise words from Lee Lozowick, the author of *Conscious Parenting* (Hohm Press, 1996):

> Trusting that the food their parents are giving them is good for them is most important for a child, and if we are constantly picking apart the food, "Oh, you know, that doesn't have your daily requirement of protein, you need your proteins, and you need your vitamins, don't forget your vitamin C, and, oh, vitamin B's, gotta have your vitamin B-12, and don't forget your calcium, and nah-nah-nah-nah-nah . . . ," we are liable to have one sick little puppy, neurotic and obsessive . . . We don't need to overeducate our children about the food they eat . . . just offer them a variety of natural, fresh healthy food and let them eat what they like of what we offer.[1]

Q. What about vitamin supplements?

A. As was discussed in Supplements and Fortified Foods in chapter two, supplements generally are unnecessary unless one or more of the following conditions exists:

1. You live in a very cloudy or northerly area so that your child is not exposed to enough sunlight for any substantial part of the year. In this case, a vitamin D supplement or foods fortified with vitamin D are highly recommended.

2. Your child is vegan or eats few eggs and dairy products. In this case, a vitamin B-12 supplement or foods fortified with B-12 are essential.

3. Your child is vegan and does not eat a substantial amount of calcium-rich foods such as green leafy vegetables and sesame-seed preparations. If that is the case, ask your child's

doctor whether a calcium supplement is warranted. If it is, make sure any calcium supplement is free of animal products and lead. Such supplements usually contain other nutrients such as magnesium, which facilitate the absorption of the calcium.

4. Your child is suffering from iron-deficiency anemia which merits an iron supplement. Unless your baby is anemic, however, an iron supplement is not necessary and may be harmful. Some obvious signs of anemia are pale skin and, in normally energetic babies, constant lack of energy. Since cows' milk does not contain significant iron, a baby who is eating and drinking a lot of dairy products to the exclusion of iron-rich foods such as green vegetables and whole grains, may develop anemia and will need an iron supplement. (*See chapters two and five for more information on iron-rich foods, and iron and dairy products.*)

5. You grow most or all of your own food, but your local soils are deficient in important minerals like iodine. Purchase some foods grown on other soils, amend your soil, and/or add appropriate supplements and fortified foods to the diet.

6. Your child is seriously ill, or for some other reason is unable to get enough of some nutrient from the offered diet to stay healthy, in which case specific supplements may be recommended by the pediatrician. Do not try to diagnose such conditions by yourself. A multi-vitamin/mineral formulated for children generally is considered safe, but supplementation beyond that should be supervised by a physician or reputable nutritionist.

Q. How should I approach our pediatrician about my baby's vegetarian diet?

A. In an ideal world, all doctors would be knowledgeable about nutrition, including vegetarian diets, but this often is not the case. Chances are that your pediatrician may not be particularly knowledgeable about vegetarianism and, therefore, may be a little wary.

The best approach is to educate yourself about sound vegetarian nutrition in as much detail as you can and to share that information with your child's doctor in a friendly way. Your confidence can inspire trust, especially when the pediatrician sees that your child is doing well.

To use a specific example: if you are told that "all babies must be given iron supplements," and your child is not anemic, suggest giving iron-rich natural foods, or small amounts of fortified foods, as an alternative. If the doctor still balks, then you need to make the ultimate decision. In choosing not to follow a doctor's directions, try not to act defensively, but instead calmly tell him or her of your decision and the reason for it. Disagreeing with the medical profession can be unpleasant, but if you have thought out what you are doing and why, and if you really are able to listen to the doctor's point of view, you should be able to make an educated decision. By talking to the doctor when you choose an alternative to his or her recommendation, you will demonstrate that a successful alternative exists, and that you are acting responsibly toward your child. And in the improbable case that difficulties do arise, he or she will have more information with which to remedy the situation.

You might find it worthwhile to search for a sympathetic doctor, especially if you live in a well-populated area. The Resources section at the end of this book contains some information on finding such a doctor.

Q. What do I do if my baby is offered meat?

A. Your reaction is an entirely personal decision, depending upon how strongly you feel about not eating meat, how much you want to shape your child's opinions, and how well you are able to respond to a meat-eating culture. If you have been able to make a vegetarian stand with your family and friends, fewer situations will arise in which your child is offered meat, at least until formal schooling begins. You may choose to strictly regulate the environment of your child until he or she is old enough to talk and think about the issue, but you cannot exert that type of control forever. Most children appear to arrive eventually at a dietary philosophy similar to their family's, just as they acquire their parents' religious beliefs and other values, but you should expect some experimentation before and during adolescence. It seems best not to interfere directly with an older child's personal exploration of this issue beyond issuing house rules and allowing open discussion without becoming judgmental.

Social and moral development are discussed in much more detail in Sharon Yntema's second book, *Vegetarian Children*. Also, keep in mind that learning to deal gracefully with difficult social situations is a valuable experience for your child, and so it is important to set a good example. The Miss Manners' etiquette books written by Judith Martin offer many amusing examples and suggestions, including some written specifically for vegetarians, which you might find useful.

Q. When should I start making sure my baby's teeth are cleaned? Are children on a vegetarian diet less likely to get cavities?

A. Cavities (dental caries) are created by prolonged exposure of the teeth to sugar. Although fluoride helps to form strong teeth that resist decay, as was discussed in chapter two, no amount of fluoride in the water or as a supplement will prevent cavities in the child who eats a lot of sugary products. Because many vegetarian foods are high in carbohydrates and sugars, vegetarian children definitely can develop cavities. Dried fruits, for example, are a natural plant food that is terrible for teeth because dried fruits are so sticky and, therefore, stay on the tooth a long time. Giving a child juice in a bottle, or allowing your child to walk around or fall asleep with a bottle of formula dangling from the mouth, also can cause rapid decay, as can frequent night nursing of an older child. The longer sugar in any form stays in contact with a tooth, the longer the active bacteria in the saliva have to produce the acid that eats away the tooth enamel and into the tooth, causing decay.

Although the bacteria that cause tooth decay (primarily *Streptococcus mutans*) thrive on sugar, you won't want to exclude any particular group of whole foods from the diet. Ideally, once teeth erupt, brushing and flossing would occur after every meal, no matter how small. That is obviously impractical, but you can improve the situation by serving regular meals, rather than allowing your child to "graze" continually, and giving your child abrasive foods after or even with sweeter foods such as dried fruits. Nuts, for example, even ground somewhat, will help remove sticky fruit, which is one reason a nut and fruit mixture is a good snack. Raw apple and crunchy vegetables such as carrots and celery also are good after-meal tooth cleansers for the child who is old enough to eat them. Finally, a good rinsing with water, which your child might even enjoy if you make it a game, can help remove food particles and reduce the amount of food coating the teeth.

Sufficient dietary calcium and magnesium are vital for producing strong and healthy teeth. This need begins before birth, since several front teeth begin to form their roots during the fourth or fifth month of pregnancy. If the supply of a number of minerals is too low in fetuses and babies, their teeth will be more susceptible to decay for the rest of their lives. In general, a healthy diet for both mother and child will promote strong teeth.

As for brushing, the American Academy of Pediatrics states, "toothbrushing by children younger than six years [should be] supervised by an adult and only a pea-sized smear of paste [should be] placed on the toothbrush beginning at two years of age."[2] Tricks to instill proper dental care habits include letting your child chew on a toothbrush while in the bathtub before bed, gently massaging the gums with a toothbrush during teething, and brushing your own teeth at the same time as your child is brushing. Some parents also use cotton to clean their baby's teeth once a day, but not all children will allow it. For further information, contact your pediatrician or a children's dentist.

Q. What about feeding a sick child?

A. Depending upon the sickness, of course, a sick child probably will not want or need many solid foods. (If your child is very ill or is losing too much weight during the course of an illness, consult your pediatrician.) Continue to offer breast milk or formula to a child who has not been weaned. Grains and legumes are often too heavy to digest for the body which is trying to heal itself. Fruit, vegetable, and sprout drinks and soups are usually much more acceptable to the sick baby, both physically and psychologically. Whole grain bread is often digested well, especially if soaked in milk or broth, and will provide strengthening nutritional value to a sick child's diet. Above all, believe your child when he or she doesn't want a lot to eat. If your child seems to be getting well but is still not eating, feed him or her small amounts of nutrient-dense foods. The less one eats, the more accustomed one becomes physically to eating small amounts, so gradually increase the amount of food you offer a child who is getting well.

Q. I have heard that milk is mucus-forming. Does this mean that I should limit the amount of milk I give my baby?

A. Dairy products do not in and of themselves create excessive mucus, but if your child appears to be producing an unusually large amount of mucus and is not sick, an allergy or food sensitivity could be the culprit. As was discussed in chapter two, except for human breast milk, dairy products are a major source of allergies, so try removing them from the diet for a week or two, and see if the problem clears up. If it does, reintroduce the dairy, and if the stuffiness returns, remove the dairy again, this time permanently. If the mucus production continues even when dairy is eliminated, another allergen might be the culprit, and you might want to consult an allergist for testing. For more information on allergies, read *Allergy Free Eating* by Liz Reno and Joanna Devrais (Celestial Arts, 1995). Also see the question on allergies, below.

Whether your child has a milk allergy or not, it is a good idea not to feed dairy products to the exclusion of other foods. Offer your child some plant-based milks, soy or nut cheeses, and calcium-rich foods such as greens and tahini. In other words, if your family is lacto-vegetarian go ahead and include cows' milk as part of the diet, but don't make it the main focus.

Q: Both my wife and I suffer from horrible allergies. How do we prevent our child from developing allergies to foods and other substances?

A: According to the American Dietetic Association, "fewer than 2 percent of adults suffer from true food allergies" and the "estimated 5 percent of children . . . with food allergies . . . usually outgrow them by the time they become adults."[3] True allergies are an immune system response to foreign substances called allergens which enter the body through the digestive and respiratory tracts or by way of the skin. Sometimes a person can have a reaction so severe it causes life-threatening anaphylactic shock, but that is rare.

Much of what people call allergies are actually food sensitivities or are caused by food-borne pathogens. Sometimes a certain food component such as lactose or gluten is not digested or metabolized well; other times a chemical, mold, or bacteria can cause an adverse reaction. So many variables are involved that it can be difficult, or even impossible, to track down the problem with any certitude. If you think you or your child is allergic or sensitive to certain foods or other substances, see an allergist for testing and advice.

As for avoiding the development of allergies and sensitivities, you will want to feed your baby according to the guidelines presented in this book. Breast-feed your child for six months. If necessary, a hypoallergenic formula can be used instead. After six months, gradually introduce solids starting with the foods least likely to cause allergies, feeding one new food every three to five days. Wait a full 12 months before introducing the following foods: dairy products, egg whites, wheat and wheat products, corn and corn products, soy products, nuts and nut products (especially peanuts), citrus fruits, and chocolate.

During lactation, the mother also might want to avoid some or all of those foods, as allergens are thought to sometimes pass into the breast milk.[4] Care must be taken to eat especially well, including the use of supplements, if such food restrictions are practiced.[5] Also note that goats' milk is not protective: one study reports that "almost 100 percent of children with confirmed CMA [cows' milk allergy] have a positive challenge with goats' milk . . ."[6]

In addition to diet, you will want to pay attention to non-food allergens and irritants such as cleaning products, dust-mites, molds, animal dander, pollens, perfumes, and tobacco smoke. Products such as HEPA-filter air purifiers and vacuum cleaners, dust mite-resistant bedding covers, and hypoallergenic cleansers can reduce the irritants your child is exposed to. Ask your allergist for details.

RESOURCES

Raising Children Toxic Free by T. Berry Brazelton, M.D., and Philip Landrigan, M.D. (Avon Books, 1994)

Q: We can't afford organic food—and there isn't much available in our area, anyway. What should we do?

A: Organically grown food has many benefits, but it is not necessarily safer or more nutritious than foods grown with modern chemical inputs. You won't want to restrict your child's access to healthy foods just because you can't buy or grow premium produce. Buy what is available, wash it well, and peel it, if possible.

Positive aspects of sustainable farming include less pollution of the air, water, and soil, which can affect the health of humans and animals both on the farm and further away—sometimes even globally. The word "sustainable" also implies that those farms will continue to be capable of producing food in the future rather than becoming so depleted they turn into virtual wastelands. Organically grown food produced locally is more likely to be picked ripe and marketed immediately, and organic farmers often choose unusual varieties which have more interesting flavors, colors, and textures than conventional ones. All of these are good reasons to choose organic foods, even without considering the direct effects specific chemical residues might have on your child's body.

The bottom line, however, is that plants cannot grow and develop normally without the substances they require, so plants grown with modern chemicals still will contain the vitamins and minerals your child needs. The exception is certain minerals such as iodine and selenium, which are deficient in some soils, but that lack will affect organic as well as conventional produce. In addition, "organic" doesn't even mean no toxic substances are used; it merely means that the substances which are used will quickly break down in the environment and won't hurt the crops or soil. Copper is an example of a very toxic substance used in organic gardening and farming.[7]

Vegetarians also must take into account that much of the fertilizer used by organic farmers comes from factory farms, feed lots, slaughterhouses, and the fishing industry. Chicken and steer manure, blood and bone meal, feathers, and fish meal, are all used by the organics industry.[8] Several well-publicized cases of food poisoning have occurred due to contamination of fruits and vegetables by animal wastes which is why it is important to wash organic produce well. If you grow your own food, consider gardening "veganically," by using organic methods and no animal products.

Q: A day care worker recently commented on our daughter's small size and hinted she might be failing to thrive because of her vegan diet. Both my husband and I are small, but we're worried that he might be right. How can we assure ourselves and others that our daughter is growing normally?

A: You need to take this seriously, not because anything is wrong with your child, but because a day care worker is in a position to report you to the authorities, even if he or she is totally mistaken —which in this situation is probably the case (*see Interacting with Others, page 116*). Failure to thrive (FTT) is a specific problem defined as "the failure to sustain a normal velocity of weight and height growth during the first three years."[9] The key words are "normal velocity." Normal is not the same as average. Normal encompasses a large range of heights and weights for any particular age group, from large to small. FTT is not a concern for a child whose weight or weight-for-height is within two standard deviations of the mean, or whose weight gain pattern has not fallen more than two standard deviations from the "previously established rate of growth."[10]

What this means is that your child can be small and still be perfectly normal, especially if that is the usual pattern in both your families. But once a growth pattern has been determined, if your child's growth deviates wildly from her original path along a given growth percentile, you will want to check with her physician to make sure nothing is wrong. If a child is diagnosed as failing to thrive, keep in mind that diet is only one facet of growth, and other problems such as illness or a genetic defect can cause retarded growth. If malnutrition is the cause, a child probably will exhibit "disproportionately low weight for height with normal head circumference," at which point not only diet, but the ability to digest and absorb food, will have to be examined.[11]

As for the concerned day care worker, talk to the director of the center and ask that all the workers be educated about vegetarian diets for children as well as the wide variations possible in normal growth. You also might have your child's pediatrician write a note for their records confirming your child's healthy growth pattern.

Conclusion

SHARON'S STORY: *Final Thoughts*

I would like to stress that there is a natural development in babies that can make a parent's job easier. If you watch carefully, you will notice that your baby will tell you what he or she needs and often can help you with the timing of introducing a spoon or a cup or finger foods or whatever the next step may be. Your responsibility as a parent is to offer nutritious, well-balanced foods, in a friendly relaxed atmosphere. George Ohsawa, who brought macrobiotics to this country, correctly implied that parents need to think about their own development in order to raise children as best they can. A parent who has made the effort to educate herself or himself adequately on vegetarian nutrition for babies, and who has spent some energy figuring out what is truly important in life and living with those principles in mind, will make a very good parent. A relaxed, healthy baby will be the natural result of such an environment.

• • •

Last Words

There you have it—a blueprint for how to raise a healthy vegetarian baby. This is an exciting time to be raising children as vegetarians. Never before has so much information been available on how to feed a child primarily or exclusively on plant foods while still providing complete nutrition. As the next century and the new millennium unfold, we undoubtedly will see many more research studies of the new generation of vegetarian babies which will confirm this choice and show even the most skeptical that it is indeed a viable one.

Feelings of love, trust, and honesty lie at the very heart of vegetarian families: love of life, and love of each other; trust in the ability of the planet to sustain and feed us, and trust in our ability to feed ourselves; and honesty about the damage we have done to that planet and the other animals and how the solution lies with us and the choices we make every day. By offering your child a well-balanced vegetarian diet, not only will you have the joy of watching your child grow and thrive, but you also will have the satisfaction of knowing you have done your utmost to teach your child sound eating habits for a healthy and humane life. In a society rife with degenerative diseases, environmental destruction, and violence, this is no small legacy to give to your child: a healthy body, a healthy mind, and a healthy soul.

Resources

Vegetarian Organizations

To find a local vegetarian society, look in your phone book, search the Internet, or contact a national vegetarian group.

The Vegetarian Resource Group
  PO Box 1463
  Baltimore, MD, 21203
  410-366-8343
  http://www.vrg.org

EarthSave International
  444 NE Ravenna Boulevard, Suite 205
  Seattle, WA 98105
  http://www.earthsave.org

The North American Vegetarian Society
  PO Box 72
  Dolgeville, NY 13329
  518-568-7970
  http://www.cyberveg.org/navs

The American Vegan Society
  PO Box H
  Malaga, NJ 08328
  609-694-2887

Vegetarian Union of North America
  PO Box 9710
  Washington, DC 20016
  http://www.ivu.org/vuna

Jewish Vegetarians of North America
    6938 Reliance Road
    Federalsburg, MD 21632
    http://www.orbyss.com/jvna.htm

Vegan.com
    http://www.vegan.com

Sci-Veg
    http://www.sci-veg.org

VegSource
    http://www.vegsource.org/

Vegetarian Awareness Network
    24-hour message: 800-USA-VEGE

Medical Practitioners

The first place to look for a medical practitioner is in the "Physicians & Surgeons, MD," section of your phone book under Family & General Practice, Obstetrics, and Pediatrics. Practitioners who understand vegetarian diets are likely also to advertise under Holistic, Nutrition, or Naturopathy as well as Chiropractic and Physicians & Surgeons, DO. Please carefully check the credentials and reputation of any professionals you contact, especially if you are entrusting them with your child's health. For further information about alternative practitioners in your area, contact the following organization:

The American Association of Naturopathic Physicians
    601 Valley Street, Suite 105
    Seattle, WA 98109
    206-298-0126
    http://www.naturopathic.org

Nutritionists

To find a nutritionist who is knowledgeable about vegetarian diets, ask your doctor for a referral or look in the phone book under

Dietitians or Nutritionists. For more information, contact the following organizations:

The American Dietetic Association
Vegetarian Nutrition Dietetic Practice Group #14
216 West Jackson Boulevard
Chicago, Illinois 60606-6995
312-899-0040
http://www.eatright.org/dpg14.html

The Society For Nutrition Education
7101 Wisconsin Avenue, Suite 901
Bethesda, MD, 20814
301-656-4938
http://www.jne.org

The American Association of Nutritional Consultants
810 S. Buffalo St.
Warsaw, IN 46580
888-828-2262
http://www.aanc.net/

Mail Order Food Companies

The following companies specialize in shipping natural food products to retail consumers:

Walnut Acres
Walnut Acres Road
Penns Creek, PA 17862
800-433-3998
http://www.walnutacres.com

Lumen Foods: The Whole Earth Vegetarian Catalog
409 Scott St.
Lake Charles, LA, 70601
800-256-2253
http://www.lumenfds.com

Indian Harvest

800-294-2433

http://www.indianharvest.com

Natural Way Mills, Inc.

Route 2, Box 37

Middle River, MN 56737

218-222-3677

Timber Crest Farms

4791 Dry Creek Road

Healdsburg, Ca 95448

707-433-8251

http://www.timbercrest.com

Phipps Beans

PO Box 349

Pescadero, CA 94060

800-279-0889

The Mail Order Catalog

PO Box 180

Summertown, TN 38483

800-695-2241

http://www.healthy-eating.com

SunOrganic Farm

PO Box 2429

Valley Center, CA 92082

888-269-9888

http://sunorganic.com

Barlean's Organic Oils

http://www.barleans.com

Endnotes

Opening Quotations

1. Benjamin Spock, MD and Steven Parker, MD, *Dr. Spock's Baby and Child Care* (Simon & Schuster, 1998), 328.
2. American Academy of Pediatrics Committee on Nutrition, *Pediatric Nutrition Handbook*, 4th ed., ed. Ronald E. Kleinman, MD (American Academy of Pediatrics, 1998), 575.
3. American Dietetic Association, Press Release: "Raising Children as Vegetarians," July 15, 1998.
4. Virginia Messina, MPH, RD and Kenneth Burke, PhD, RD, "Position of the American Dietetic Association: Vegetarian Diets," ADA website (http://www. eatright.org), 1998.
5. Linda Gay, RD, *The Yale Guide to Children's Nutrition*, ed. William V. Tamborlane, MD (Yale University Press, 1997), 84.
6. Robert Garrison, RPh and Elizabeth Somer, RD, *The Nutrition Desk Reference* (Keats Publishing, 1995), 588.
7. Virginia Messina, MPH, RD and Mark Messina, PhD, *The Vegetarian Way* (Three Rivers Press, 1996), 1.
8. Reply to a letter on NUTRIQUEST, a service of the Cornell University Division of Nutritional Sciences. Cornell University website (http://www.cornell.edu), 1998.
9. William Harris, MD, author of *The Scientific Basis of Vegetarianism*, as quoted on his website on VegSource (http://www.vegsource. edu).
10. Gill Langley, MA, PhD, MIBiol, *Vegan Nutrition* (Vegan Society, United Kingdom, 1995), 165–166.
11. *Nutrition and Your Health: Dietary Guidelines for Americans*, 1995.

Chapter One

1. D. B. Jelliffe, "Infant Nutrition in the Subtropics and Tropics," *World Health Organization Monograph Series 29* (Geneva: World Health Organization, 1955), 122.
2. Harvey Diamond, *Fit for Life II: Living Health* (Warner Books, 1987), 269.
3. Dixie Farley, "More People Trying Vegetarian Diets," *FDA Consumer*, FDA website (http://www.fda.gov), October 1995 with revisions made in January 1996.
4. J. M. O'Connell, M. J. Dibley, et al., "Growth of Vegetarian Children: The Farm Study," *Pediatrics* 84, no. 3 (1989): 475–481.

5. Rupert Fike, ed., *Voices from The Farm: Adventures in Community Living* (Book Publishing Company, 1998), xi.

6. The Farm website (http://www.thefarm.org), 1999.

7. O'Connell, et al.

8. *Ibid.*, 480.

9. Ellen G. White, *Sanitarium Dietary: Counsels on Diet and Foods* (Hagerstown, MD: Review and Herald Publishing Association, 1976), 294.

10. Calvary Community Church website (http://www.calvarycommunity.com), 1998.

11. Loma Linda University website (http://www.llu.edu), 1998.

12. The National Institute of Nutrition (Canada), "Risks and Benefits of Vegetarian Diets," *Nutrition Today* (March/April 1990): 27–29.

13. B. M. Anderson, R. S. Gibson, and J. H. Sabry, "The iron and zinc status of long-term vegetarian women," *The American Journal of Clinical Nutrition* 34 (1981): 1042–1048.

14. J. Sabaté, K. D. Linsted, R. D. Harris, and A. Sánchez, "Attained height of lacto-ovo vegetarian children and adolescents," *European Journal of Clinical Nutrition* 45 (1991): 51–58.

15. J. Sabaté, M. C. Llorca, and A. Sánchez, "Lower height of lacto-ovo vegetarian girls at preadolescence: An indicator of physical maturation delay?" *Journal of the American Dietetic Association* 92, no. 10 (1992): 1263–1264.

16. S. F. Knutsen, "Lifestyle and the use of health services," *American Journal of Clinical Nutrition* 59 suppl. (1994): 1171S–1175S.

17. G. E. Fraser, "Determinants of ischemic heart disease in Seventh-day Adventists: a review," *American Journal of Clinical Nutrition* 48 (1988): 833–836.

18. F. A. Tylavsky and J. J. B. Anderson, "Dietary factors in bone health of elderly lacto-ovo vegetarian and omnivorous women," *American Journal of Clinical Nutrition* 48 (1988): 842–849.

19. I. S. Hunt, N. J. Murphy, and C. Henderson, "Food and nutrient intake of Seventh-day Adventist women," *American Journal of Clinical Nutrition* 48 (1988): 850–851.

20. L. J. Beilin, "Vegetarian and other complex diets, fats, fiber, and hypertension," *American Journal of Clinical Nutrition* 59 suppl. (1994): 1130S–1135S.

21. P. K. Mills, W. L. Beeson, R. L. Phillips, and G. E. Fraser, "Cancer incidence among California Seventh-day Adventists, 1976–1982," *American Journal of Clinical Nutrition* 59 suppl. (1994): 1136S–1142S.

22. V. Fønnebø, "The healthy Seventh-day Adventist lifestyle: what is the Norwegian experience?" *American Journal of Clinical Nutrition* 59 suppl. (1994): 1124S–1129S.23.

23. George Ohsawa, *Zen Macrobiotics* (Ohsawa Foundation, 1971), 82.

24. *Ibid.*, 40.

25. Edward Esko, *Basics and Benefits of Macrobiotics: Essays on the*

Macrobiotic Way of Personal and Planetary Health (One Peaceful World Press, 1995). From book excerpt published on Macrobiotics Online website (http://www.macrobiotics.org).

26. Michio Kushi, *The Macrobiotic Way* (Avery Publishing Group, 1993), 28–31.

27. "Inadequate vegan diets at weaning," *Nutrition Reviews* 48, no. 8 (1990): 323–325.

28. P. C. Dagnelie, W. A. van Staveren, "Macrobiotic nutrition and child health: results of a population-based, mixed-longitudinal cohort study in The Netherlands," *American Journal of Clinical Nutrition* 59 suppl. (1994): 1187S–1196S.

29. B. L. Specker, "Nutritional concerns of lactating women consuming vegetarian diets," *American Journal of Clinical Nutrition* 59 suppl. (1994): 1182S–1186S.

30. W. A. van Staveren and P. C. Dagnelie, "Food consumption, growth, and development of Dutch children fed on alternative diets," *American Journal of Clinical Nutrition* 48 (1988): 819–821.

31. P. C. Dagnelie, W. A. van Staveren, et al., "Nutrients and contaminants in human milk from mothers on macrobiotic and ominvorous diets," *European Journal of Clinical Nutrition* 46 (1992): 355–366.

32. D. R. Miller, B. L. Specker, M. L. Ho, and E. J. Norman, "Vitamin B-12 status in a macrobiotic community," *American Journal of Clinical Nutrition* 53 (1991): 524–529.

33. P. C. Dagnelie, W. A. van Staveren, et al., "High prevalence of rickets in infants on macrobiotic diets," *American Journal of Clinical Nutrition* 51 (1990): 202–208.

34. M. Van Dusseldorp, I. C. W. Arts, et al., "Catch-up growth in children fed a macrobiotic diet in early childhood," *The Journal of Clinical Nutrition* 126, no. 12 (1996): 2977–2983.

35. Michio Kushi and Aveline Kushi with Edward Esko and Wendy Esko, *Raising Healthy Kids* (Avery Publishing Group, 1994), 78.

36. S. M. Asser and R. Swan, "Child Fatalities from Religion-Motivated Medical Neglect," *Pediatrics* 101, no. 4 (1998): 625–629.

37. Society for the Promotion of Buddhism, *The Teaching of Buddha* (Tokyo, Japan, 1966), 32.

38. The China-Cornell-Oxford Project Division of Nutritional Sciences, Cornell University website (http://www.cornell.edu), 1998.

39. T. C. Campbell and C. Junshi, "Diet and chronic degenerative diseases: perspectives from China," *American Journal of Clinical Nutrition* 59 suppl. (1994): 1153S–1161S.

40. The Laws of Manu V, Hindu text, as quoted in *The Extended Circle: A Commonplace Book of Animal Rights*, ed. Jon Wynne-Tyson (Paragon House, 1985), 122.

41. As quoted in *The Extended Circle*, 140.

42. Jaffrey Madhur, *World-of-the-East Vegetarian Cookbook* (Alfred A. Knopf, 1987).

43. T. A. B. Sanders and S. Reddy, "Vegetarian diets and children," *American Journal of Clinical Nutrition* 59 suppl. (1994): 1176S–1181S.

44. S. Reddy and T. A. B. Sanders, "Haematological studies on premenopausal Indian and Caucasian vegetarians compared with Caucasian omnivores," *British Journal of Nutrition* 64 (1990): 331–338.

45. J. R. Hebert, "Relationship of vegetarianism to child growth in South India," *The American Journal of Clinical Nutrition* 42 (1985): 1246–1254.

46. Rudolph M. Ballentine, MD, *Diet & Nutrition: A Holistic Approach* (Himalayan Institute, 1978), 424–425.

47. Soie Yoneda, *Zen Vegetarian Cooking* (Kodansha, 1998), 33.

48. K. Cwiertka, "A note on the making of culinary tradition—an example of modern Japan," *Appetite* 30, no. 2 (1998): 117–128.

49. C. Nagata, N. Takatsuka, Y. Kurisu, and H. Shimizu, "Decreased serum total cholesterol concentration is associated with high intake of soy products in Japanese men and women," *Journal of Nutrition* 128, no. 2 (1998): 209–213.

50. C. Nagata, N. Takatsuka, S. Inaba, N. Kawakami, and H. Shimizu, "Effect of soymilk consumption on serum estrogen concentrations in premenopausal Japanese women," *Journal of the National Cancer Institute* 90, no. 23 (1998): 1830–1835.

51. K. Nakachi, K. Suemasu, K. Suga, T. Takeo, K. Imai, and Y. Higashi, "Influence of drinking green tea on breast cancer malignancy among Japanese patients," *Japanese Journal of Cancer Research* 89, no. 3 (1998): 254–261.

52. K. Imai, K. Suga, and K. Nakachi, "Cancer-preventive effects of drinking green tea among a Japanese population," *Preventive Medicine* 26, no. 6 (1997): 769–775.

53. T. Hirohata and S. Kono, "Diet/nutrition and stomach cancer in Japan," *International Journal of Cancer* suppl 10 (1997): 34–36.

54. T. Kitagawa, M. Owada, T. Urakimi, and K. Yamauchi, "Increased incidence of non-insulin dependent diabetes mellitus among Japanese schoolchildren correlates with an increased intake of animal protein and fat," *Clinical Pediatrics* 37, no. 2 (1998): 111–115.

55. Kristine Emiko Iwasaki, interview with Christine Beard, 1998.

56. Terry Shintani, MD, JD, MPH, Hawaii Diet website (http://www.hawaiidiet.com), 1998.

57. Lecture by Dr. Terry Shintani, attended by Christine Beard, "Plant-based Nutrition Throughout the Life Cycle" (Health Care Conference, EarthSave Taste of Health Festival, Seattle, WA, 1998).

58. T. T. Shintani, C. K. Hughes, S. Beckham, and H. K. O'Connor, "Obesity and cardiovascular risk intervention through the ad libitum feeding of traditional Hawaiian diet," *American Journal of Clinical Nutrition* 53 suppl. (1991): 1647S–1651S.

59. T. T. Shintani, S. Bećkham, H. K. O'Connor, C. Hughes, and A. Sato, "The Waianae Diet Program: a culturally sensitive, community-based

obesity and clinical intervention program for the Native Hawaiian population," *Hawaii Medical Journal* 53, no. 5 (1994): 136–141, 147.

60. Terry Shintani, MD, JD, MPH, Hawaii Diet website.

61. "Isles of Hiva: Life of the Land," Polynesian Voyaging Society website (http://leahi.kcc.hawaii.edu/org/pvs/), 1999.

62. *Ibid.*

63. Sally De Vore and Thelma White, *The Appetites of Man* (Doubleday, 1978), 16.

64. World Health Organization, "Micronutrient malnutrition," *World Health*, 50th year, no. 4 (1997): 38.

65. D. B. Jelliffe, *Infant Nutrition in the Subtropics and Tropics* (World Health Organization Monograph Series 29, 1955), 7.

66. *Ibid.*, 122.

67. *Ibid.*, 27.

68. *Ibid.*, 30.

69. *Ibid.*, 159.

70. *Ibid.*, 137.

71. *Indian Council of Medical Research, Studies on Weaning and Supplementary Foods* (Indian Council of Medical Research, 1974), 2.

72. *Ibid.*, 14.

73. *Ibid.*, preface.

74. K. M. Hendricks, and S. H. Badruddin, "Weaning Recommendations: The Scientific Basis," *Nutrition Reviews* 50, no. 5 (1992): 125–133.

75. World Health Organization, *Weaning from breast milk to family food: A guide for health and community workers* (1988).

76. M. Cameron and Y. Hofvander, *Manual on feeding infants and young children*, 3rd ed. (Oxford Medical Publications, 1990).

77. J. Nemerofsky, "The Black Hebrews (abstract)," *Society* 32, no. 1 (1994): 72.

78. E. D. Shinwell and R Gorodischer, "Totally vegetarian diets and infant nutrition," *Pediatrics* 70, no. 4 (1982): 582–586.

79. C. Jacobs and J. T. Dwyer, "Vegetarian children: appropriate and inappropriate diets," *American Journal of Clinical Nutrition* 48 (1988): 811–818.

80. F. Renault, P. Verstichel, J. Ploussard, and J Costil, "Neuropathy in two cobalamin-deficient breast-fed infants of vegetarian mothers," *Muscle & Nerve* 22, no. 2 (1999): 252–254.

81. T. A. B. Sanders, "Growth and development of British vegan children," *American Journal of Clinical Nutrition* 48 (1988): 822–825.

82. J. T. Dwyer, "Health aspects of vegetarian diets," *American Journal of Clinical Nutrition* 48 (1988): 712–738.

83. The National Institute of Nutrition (Canada), "Risks and Benefits of Vegetarian Diets," *Nutrition Today* (March/April 1990): 27–29.

84. J. T. Dwyer, "Vegetarian eating patterns: science, values, and food choices—where do we go from here?" *American Journal of Clinical Nutrition* 59 suppl. (1994): 1255S–1262S.

Chapter Two

1. Lloyd Biggle, Jr., *The Light That Never Was* (DAW, 1973), as quoted in *The Extended Circle*, ed. Jon Wynne-Tyson (Paragon House, 1989), 22.

2. *Food Safety and Inspection Service, Meat and Poultry Product Recalls*, USDA website (http://www.usda.gov), updated January 11, 1999.

3. M. E. Potter, Y. Motarjemi, and F. K. Käferstein. "Emerging foodborne diseases," *World Health* 50th year, no. 1 (1997): 16–17.

4. F. X. Meslin, K. Stöhr, and P. Formenty, "Emerging zoonoses," *World Health* 50th year, no. 1 (1997): 18–19.

5. J. D. Gussow, "Ecology and vegetarian considerations: does environmental responsibility demand the elimination of livestock?" *American Journal of Clinical Nutrition* 59 suppl. (1994): 1110S–1116S.

6. S. Lewis. An opinion on the global impact of meat consumption. *American Journal of Clinical Nutrition* 59 suppl (1994): 1099S–1102S.

7. Peggy Pipes, *Nutrition in Infancy and Childhood* (Mosby, 1977), 1.

8. National Academy of Sciences, Recommended Dietary Allowances (National Institute of Health, 1974), 1.

9. NRC/NAS' Recommended Dietary Allowances, December 8, 1989, FDA website (http://www.fda.gov).

10. A. A. Yates, S. A. Schlicker, and C. W. Suitor, "Dietary Reference Intakes: The new basis for recommendations for calcium and related nutrients, B vitamins, and choline," *Journal of the American Dietetic Association* 98, no. 6 (1998): 699–706.

11. National Academy of Sciences, Recommended Dietary Allowances, 2.

12. *Ibid.*, 86.

13. La Leche League International, The Womanly Art of Breastfeeding (PLUME, 1997), 339.

14. *The Yale Guide to Children's Nutrition*, ed. William V. Tamborlane, MD (Yale University Press, 1997), 211–214.

15. *Ibid.*, 231.

16. Gil Langley, MA, PhD, MIBiol, *Vegan Nutrition* (Vegan Society, 1995), 130.

17. National Academy of Sciences, Recommended Dietary Allowances, 41.

18. Robert Garrison, MA, RPh and Elizabeth Somer, MA, RD, *The Nutrition Desk Reference* (Keats Publishing, 1995), 39–42.

19. The American Society for Nutritional Sciences website (http://www.nutrition.org), 1998.

20. American Academy of Pediatrics Committee on Nutrition, "Soy Protein-based Formulas: Recommendations for Use in Infant Feeding," *Pediatrics* 101, no. 1 (1998): 148–152.

21. Mark Messina, PhD and Virginia Messina, MPH, RD, *The Dietitian's Guide to Vegetarian Diets: Issues and Applications* (Aspen Publishers, 1996), 86.

22. Langley, *Vegan Nutrition*, 7.

23. Messina and Messina, *The Dietitian's Guide to Vegetarian Diets*, 109–122.

24. Garrison and Somer, *The Nutrition Desk Reference*, 241.

25. Virginia Messina, MPH, RD and Mark Messina, PhD, *The Vegetarian Way: Total Health for You and Your Family* (Three Rivers Press, 1996), 184.

26. Messina and Messina, *The Dietitian's Guide to Vegetarian Diets*, 87.

27. G. J. Nelson, "Dietary fat, trans fatty acids, and risk of coronary heart disease," *Nutrition Reviews* 56, no. 8 (1988): 250–252.

28. D.P. Rose, "Dietary fats and cancer," *American Journal of Clinical Nutrition* 66 suppl. (1997): 998S–1003S.

29. C. L. Rock, et al., "Bioavailability of ß-Carotene is lower in raw than processed carrots and spinach in women," *Journal of Nutrition* 128 (1998): 913–916.

30. Messina and Messina, *The Dietitian's Guide to Vegetarian Diets*, 180.

31. R. Namgung, R. D. Tsang, C. Lee, et al., "Low total body bone mineral content and high bone resorption in Korean winter-born versus summer-born newborn infants," *The Journal of Pediatrics* 132, no. 3 (1998): 421–424.

32. M. J. Park, R. Namgung, D. H. Kim, and R. C. Tsang, "Bone mineral content is not reduced despite low vitamin D status in breast milk-fed infants versus cow's milk based formula-fed infants," *The Journal of Pediatrics* 132, no. 4 (1998): 641–645.

33. Messina and Messina, *The Dietitian's Guide to Vegetarian Diets*, 180.

34. G. M. Johnson, "Powdered goat's milk: pyridoxine deficiency and status epilepticus," *Clinical Pediatrics* 21, no. 8 (August 1982): 494–495.

35. J. A. Halsted, J. Carroll, and S. Robert, "Serum and tissue concentrations of vitamin B-12 in certain pathologic states," *New England Journal of Medicine* 260 (1959): 575–580.

36. P. C. Dagnelie, W. A. van Staveren, and H. van den Berg, "Vitamin B-12 from algae appears not to be bioavailable," *American Journal of Clinical Nutrition* 53 (1991): 695–697.

37. Rauma, et. al., Letter to the Editor, *The Journal of Nutrition* 127, no. 2 (1997): 380.

38. Garrison and Somer, *The Nutrition Desk Reference*, 147.

39. Virginia Messina, MPH, RD and Kenneth Burke, PhD, RD, "Position of the American Dietetic Association: Vegetarian Diets," ADA website (http://www.eatright.org), 1998.

40. Garrison and Somer, *The Nutrition Desk Reference*, 150.

41. Messina and Messina, *The Dietitian's Guide to Vegetarian Diets*, 100.

42. *Ibid.*, 100.

43. Scott Van Why and Lisa Devine, The Yale Guide to Children's Nutrition, ed. William Tamborlane, MD (Yale University Press, 1987), 246.

44. Vesanto Melina, RD, Brenda Davis, RD, and Victoria Harrison, RD, *Becoming Vegetarian: The Complete Guide to Adopting a Healthy Vegetarian Diet* (Book Publishing Company, 1995), 108.

45. R. H. Seiwitz, R. E. Nowjack-Raymer, A. Kingman, and W. S. Driscoll, "Dental caries and dental flourosis among schoolchildren who were lifelong residents of communities having either low or optimal levels of fluoride in drinking water," *Journal of Public Health Dentistry* 58, no. 1 (1998): 28–35.

46. Eliana V. M. Borigato and Francisco E. Martinez, "Iron nutritional status is improved in Brazilian preterm infants fed food cooked in iron pots," *Journal of Nutrition* 128 (1998): 855.

47. Alice C. Yao, MD and John Lind, MD, *Placental Transfusion: A Clinical and Physiological Study* (Charles C. Thomas Publisher, 1982).

48. Messina and Messina, *The Vegetarian Way*, 186.

49. Borigato and Martinez, 855–859.

50. J. Park and H. C. Brittin, "Increased iron content of food due to stainless steel cookware," *Journal of the American Dietetic Association* 97, no. 6 (1997): 659–661.

51. Messina and Messina, *The Dietitian's Guide to Vegetarian Diets*, 128.

52. "Biomedicine: Can selenium avert prostate cancer?" *Science News* d154, no. 12 (1998): 188.

53. Messina and Messina, *The Dietitian's Guide to Vegetarian Diets*, 138.

54. *Ibid.*, 132.

55. American Academy of Pediatrics Committee on Nutrition, Pediatric Nutrition Handbook, 4th ed., ed. Ronald E. Kleinman, MD (American Academy of Pediatrics, 1998), 580.

56. Garrison and Somer, *The Nutrition Desk Reference*, 217.

57. G. E. Fraser, "Diet and coronary heart disease: beyond dietary fats and low-density-lipoprotein cholesterol," *American Journal of Clinical Nutrition* 59 suppl. (1994): 1117S–1123S.

58. K. D. Setchell, L. Zimmer-Nechemias, J. Cai, and J. E. Heubi, "Exposure of infants to phyto-oestrogens from soy-based infant formula," *Lancet* 350 (July 1997): 23–27.

59. *Ibid.*

60. J. W. Anderson, B. M. Smith, and N. J. Gustafson, "Health benefits and practical aspects of high-fiber diets," *American Journal of Clinical Nutrition* 59 suppl. (1994): 1242S–1247S.

61. Andrew Weil, MD, *Eight Weeks to Optimal Health* (Alfred A. Knopf, 1997), 64–65.

62. Benjamin Spock, MD and Steven J. Parker, MD, *Dr. Spock's Baby and Child Care* (Simon & Schuster, 1998), 169–170.

63. Vegetarian Research Group 1997 Roper Poll, "How Many Vegetarians Are There?" *Vegetarian Journal* 16, no. 5 (1997), *Vegetarian Journal* excerpts, Vegetarian Resource Group website (http://www.vrg. org).

64. P. A. Stehr-Green, J. C. Wohlleb, W. Royce, and S. L. Head, "An evaluation of serum pesticide residue levels and liver function in persons exposed to dairy products contaminated with heptachlor," (Second National Health and Nutrition Examination Survey, NHANES). *The Journal of the American Medical Association* 259, no. 3 (1988): 374.

65. V. L. Olejer, "Food hypersensitivities," in *Handbook of Pediatric Nutrition*, ed. P. M. Queen and C. E. Lang (Aspen Publishing, 1993), 206–231.

66. T. Decsi, V. Veitl, and I. Burus, "Plasma amino acid concentrations, indexes of protein metabolism and growth in healthy, full-term infants fed partially hydrolyzed infant formula," *Journal of Pediatric Gastroenterology and Nutrition* 27, no. 1 (1998): 12–16.

67. G. Iacono, F. Cavataio, et al., "Intolerance of cow's milk and chronic constipation in children," *New England Journal of Medicine* 339 (1998): 16.

68. E. E. Telzak, L.D. Budnick, M. S. Z. Greenberg, et al., "A nosocomial outbreak of Salmonella enteritidis infection due to the consumption of raw eggs," *New England Journal of Medicine* 323, no. 6 (1990): 394.

69. With permission from Dr. Harris, from a statement made on the Sci-Veg website (http://www.sci-veg.com), 1998.

70. Messina and Messina, *The Dietitian's Guide to Vegetarian Diets*, 181.

71. American Society for Nutritional Sciences website (http://www.nutrition.org), 1998.

72. Values obtained from the National Academy of Sciences website (http://www.nas.edu), 1998.

73. Yates, et al., "Dietary Reference Intakes," 701.

74. The United States Department of Agriculture, *Composition of Foods Handbook No. 8.*

Chapter Three

1. Wendell Berry, as quoted in *The One-Straw Revolution* (Rodale Press, 1978).

2. T. A. B. Sanders and S. Reddy, "The influence of a vegetarian diet on the fatty acid composition of human milk and the essential fatty acid status of the infant," *Department of Nutritional Dietetics* 120 (1992): S71–S77.

3. B. Davis, "Essential fatty acids in vegetarian nutrition," *Issues in Vegetarian Dietetics* (Summer 1998): 5–7.

4. B. Koletzko, I. Thiel, and S. Springer, "Lipids in human milk: a model for infant formula?" *European Journal of Clinical Nutrition* 46 suppl. (1992): 45S–55S.

5. T. K. Jones, B. M. Lawson, "Profound neonatal congestive heart failure caused by maternal consumption of blue cohosh herbal medication," *The Journal of Pediatrics* 132, no. 4 (1998): 550–552.

6. "Medical Journal Cites Harm from Herbal Remedies," *San Francisco Chronicle/New York Times*, September 17, 1998.

7. Mark Messina, PhD and Virginia Messina, MPH, RD, *The Dietitian's Guide to Vegetarian Diets: Issues and Applications* (Aspen Publishers, 1996), 247.

8. *Ibid.*, 250.

9. E. Raum, et al., "Contamination of human breast milk with organochlorine residues: a comparison between East and West Germany through sentinel practice networks," *Journal of Epidemiology & Community Health* 52 suppl 1 (1998): 50S–55S.

10. U.S. Department of Health and Human Services, Maternal and Child Health Bureau, DHHS Publication No. HRSA-M-DSEA-96-5 (Washington, D.C.: GPO, September 1996), 20.

11. *Ibid.*, 20.

12. Charles R. Attwood, MD, *A Vegetarian Doctor Speaks Out* (Hohm Press, 1998), 157–158.

13. *Ibid.*,159–161.

14. Shirley Dumas, personal interview with Christine Beard, 1998.

15. Steven P. Shelov and Robert E. Hannemann, eds., *Caring for Your Baby and Young Child: Birth to Age 5*, rev. ed. (The American Academy of Pediatrics, 1998), 122.

16. *Ibid.*, 30–31.

17. Values obtained from the National Academy of Sciences website (http://www.nas.edu), 1998.

18. A. A. Yates, et al., "Dietary Reference Intakes: The new basis for recommendations for calcium and related nutrients, B vitamins, and choline," *Journal of the American Dietetic Association* 98, no. 6 (1998): 701.

Chapter Four

1. Rebecca F. Black, Leasa Jarman, and Jan B. Simpson, *The Management of Breastfeeding, Lactation Specialist Self-Study Series: Module 4* (Jones and Bartlett, 1998), 11.

2. American Academy of Pediatrics Committee on Nutrition, *Pediatric Nutrition Handbook*, 4th ed., ed. Ronald E. Kleinman, MD, (American Academy of Pediatrics, 1998), 89.

3. Black, et al., *The Management of Breastfeeding*, 15.

4. *Pediatric Nutrition Handbook*, 89–90.

5. Black, et al., *The Management of Breastfeeding*, 8

6. K. M. Hendricks and S. H. Badruddin, "Weaning Recommendations: The Scientific Basis," *Nutrition Reviews* 50, no. 5 (1992): 125–133.

7. *Pediatric Nutrition Handbook*, 91.

8. *Ibid.*, 96–99.

9. Hendricks and Badruddin.

10. Hendricks and Badruddin.

11. *Pediatric Nutrition Handbook*, 92–96.
12. *Ibid.*, 90.
13. *Ibid.*, 98.
14. Hendricks and Badruddin.
15. Hendricks and Badruddin.
16. *Pediatric Nutrition Handbook*, 91.
17. *Ibid.*, 92.
18. Hendricks and Badruddin.
19. *Pediatric Nutrition Handbook*, 99–100.
20. J. S. Forsyth, "Is it worthwhile breast-feeding?" *European Journal of Clinical Nutrition* 46 suppl. (1992): 19S–25S.
21. A. S. Goldman, S. Chheda, and R. Garofalo, "Evolution of immunologic functions of the mammary gland and the postnatal development of immunity," *Pediatric Research* 43, no. 2 (1998): 155–162.
22. P. J. Kling, et al., "Human milk as a potential enteral source of erythropoietin," *Pediatric Research* 43, no. 2 (1998): 216–221.
23. Black, et al., *Management of Breastfeeding*, 15.
24. Hendricks and Badruddin.
25. *Ibid.*
26. Christine Repault, *Children's Gastronomique* (Crown Publications, 1968), 372.
27. William Harris, MD, *The Scientific Basis of Vegetarianism* (Hawaii Health Publishers, 1996), 77.
28. R. J. Kuczmarski, "Revised growth charts due in late 1998," *AAP NEWS* 14, no. 9 (1998).
29. J. Sabaté, M. C. Llorca, and A. Sánchez, "Lower height of lacto-ovo vegetarian girls at preadolescence: An indicator of physical maturation delay?" *Journal of the American Dietetic Association* 92, no. 10 (1992): 1263–1264.
30. S. Chinn, R. J. Rona, M. C. Guilliford, and J. Hammond, "Weight-for-height in children aged 4-12 years. A new index compared to the normalized body mass index," *European Journal of Clinical Nutrition* 46 (1992): 489–500.
31. Kuczmarski.
32. *Ibid.*
33. T. A. B. Sanders and S. Reddy, "Vegetarian diets and children," *American Journal of Clinical Nutrition* 59 suppl. (1994): 1176S–1181S.
34. J. Sabaté, K. D. Linsted, R. D. Harris, and A. Sánchez, "Attained height of lacto-ovo vegetarian children and adolescents," *European Journal of Clinical Nutrition* 45 (1991): 51–58.
35. Kuczmarski.

Chapter Five

1. Christine Repault, *Children's Gastronomique* (Crown Publications, 1968), 8.

2. M. Delahoyde, S. C. Despenich, "Creating meat-eaters: the child as advertising target," *Journal of Popular Culture* 28, no. 1 (1994): 135–150.

3. Massanobu Fukuoka, *The One-Straw Revolution* (Rodale Press, 1978), 140–141.

4. Michael Klaper, MD, *Pregnancy, Children, and the Vegan Diet* (Gentle World, 1988), 49.

5. Virginia Messina, MPH, RD and Mark Messina, PhD, *The Vegetarian Way: Total Health for You and Your Family* (Three Rivers Press, 1996), 187.

6. Benjamin Spock, MD and Steven Parker, MD, *Dr. Spock's Baby and Child Care* (Simon & Schuster, 1998), 193.

7. Mark Messina, PhD and Virginia Messina, MPH, RD, *The Dietitian's Guide to Vegetarian Diets: Issues and Applications* (Aspen Publishers, 1996), 264.

8. G. P. Savage, "Nutritional value of sprouted mung beans," *Nutrition Today* (May/June 1990): 21–24.

9. Steve Meyerowitz, "Sprout Man, Raw Foodist," *Vegetarian Times* (August 1979): 26.

10. *Pediatric Nutrition Handbook*, 131–132.

11. "The Bitter Truth: Do Some People Inherit a Distaste for Broccoli?" *Science News* 152 (July 12, 1997): 24–25.

Chapter Six

1. Altman, Nathaniel, *Eating for Life* (Theosophical Publishing House, 1977) 28. Quoted with permission of the publisher.

2. Charles Attwood, MD, *A Vegetarian Doctor Speaks Out* (Hohm Press, 1998), 13–14.

3. Steven P. Shelov and Robert E. Hannemann, eds. *Caring for Your Baby and Young Child: Birth to Age 5*, rev. ed. (The American Academy of Pediatrics, 1998), 154.

4. U.S. Department of Health & Human Services, Child Health USA '95, Publication No. HRSA-M-DSEA-96-5 (Washington, D.C.: GPO, September 1996), 29.

5. Ruth Lawrence, MD, spokeswoman for the American Academy of Pediatrics, as quoted by Rebecca D. Williams, "Breast-Feeding Best Bet for Babies," *FDA Consumer* (October 1995).

6. Benjamin Spock, MD and Steven Parker, MD, *Dr. Spock's Baby and Child Care* (Simon & Schuster, 1998), 103.

7. Donna Caseria, Barbara Ackerman, and Brian Forsyth, *The Yale Guide to Children's Nutrition*, 38–39.

8. Spock and Parker, 140.

9. H. L. Greene, P. Porchelli, E. Adcock, and L. Swift, "Vitamins for newborn infant formulas: a review of recommendations with emphasis on data from low birth-weight infants," *European Journal of Clinical Nutrition* 46 suppl.4 (1992): 1S–8S.

10. Mark Messina, PhD and Virginia Messina, MPH, RD, *The Dietitian's Guide to Vegetarian Diets: Issues and Applications* (Aspen Publishers, 1996), 263.
11. American Academy of Pediatrics Committee on Nutrition, *Pediatric Nutrition Handbook*, 4th ed., ed. Ronald E. Kleinman, MD (American Academy of Pediatrics, 1998), 45.
12. Dr. Clara M. Davis, "Results of the Self-Selection of Diets by Young Children," *Child and Family*, 10, no. 3 (1971): 217.
13. Elisabeth A. Reilly and Nancy A. Held, *The Yale Guide to Children's Nutrition*, 46.

Chapter Seven

1. Lee Lozowick, *Conscious Parenting* (Hohm Press, 1997), 317–318.
2. American Academy of Pediatrics Committee on Nutrition, *Pediatric Nutrition Handbook*, 4th ed., ed. Ronald E. Kleinman, MD (American Academy of Pediatrics, 1998), 525.
3. Roberta Larson Duyff, *The American Dietetic Association's Complete Food & Nutrition Guide* (Chronimed Publishing, 1998), 203.
4. Y. Fukushima, Y. Kawata, T. Onda, and M. Kitagawa, "Consumption of cow milk and egg by lactating women and the presence of beta-lactoglobulin and ovalbumin in breast milk," *American Journal of Clinical Nutrition* 65, no. 1 (1997): 30–35.
5. D. W. Hide, "Prophylaxis of allergic disease—is it worthwhile?" *European Journal of Clinical Nutrition* 46 suppl. 4 (1992): 21S–28S.
6. B. L. Bruno, "Prophylaxis of cow's milk allergy," *Pediatric Allergy and Immunology* 8 suppl. 10 (1997): 11S–15S.
7. California Certified Organic Farmers: Certification Standards, CCOF Website (http://www.ccof.org), 1999.
8. *Ibid.*
9. *Pediatric Nutrition Handbook*, 325.
10. *Ibid.*, 325.
11. *Ibid.*, 327.

Bibliography

A'o, Lono Kahuna Kupua. *Don't Drink the Water: The Essential Guide to Our Contaminated Drinking Water and What You Can Do About It.* Kali Press, 1996.

Akers, Keith. *A Vegetarian Sourcebook.* Vegetarian Press, 1993.

Attwood, Charles. *Dr. Attwood's Low-Fat Prescription for Kids.* Viking, 1995.

_____. *A Vegetarian Doctor Speaks Out.* Hohm Press, 1998.*

Black, Rebecca F.; Jarman, Leasa; and Simpson, Jan B., *The Science of Breast-feeding, Lactation Specialist Self-Study Series: Module 3.* Jones and Bartlett Publishers, 1998.

_____. *The Management of Breast-feeding, Lactation Specialist Self-Study Series: Module 4.* Jones and Bartlett Publishers, 1998.

The Boston Women's Health Book Collective. *Our Bodies, Ourselves: for the New Century.* Simon & Schuster, 1998.

Bumilligarner, Marlene Anne; and Roy, Johanna (Illustrator). *The New Book of Whole Grains: More Than 200 Recipes Featuring Whole Grains, Including Amaranth, Quinoa, Wheat, Spelt, Oats, Rye, Barley, and Millet.* St. Martin's Griffin, 1997.

Dodt, Colleen K. *Natural Baby Care: Pure and Soothing Recipes and Techniques for Mothers and Babies.* Storey Communications, 1997.

Duyff, Roberta Larson. *The American Dietetic Association's Complete Food & Nutrition Guide.* Chronimed Publishing, 1998.

Erasmus, Udo. *Fats that Heal, Fats That Kill: The Complete Guide to Fats, Oils, Cholesterol and Human Health.* Alive Books, 1993.

Fike, Rupert, ed. *Voices from the Farm: Adventures in Community Living.* Book Publishing Company, 1998.

Ford, Marjorie Winn; Hillyard, Susan; and Koock, Mary Faulk. *The Deaf Smith Country Cookbook: Natural Foods for Family Kitchens.* Collier Books, Macmillan Publishing, 1973.

Garrison, Robert; and Somer, Elizabeth. *The Nutrition Desk Reference.* Keats Publishing, 1995.

Hagler, Louise; and Bates, Dorothy R; eds. *The New Farm Vegetarian Cookbook.* Book Publishing Company, 1988.

Harris, William. *The Scientific Basis of Vegetarianism.* Hawaii Health Publishers, 1996.

Hirschmann, Jane R.; and Zaphiropoulos, Lela. *Preventing Childhood Eating Problems: A Practical, Positive Approach to Raising Kids*

Free of Food & Weight Conflicts. Gurze Designs & Books, 1993.

Hurd, Frank J.; and Hurd, Rosalie. *Ten Talents.* The College Press, 1985.

Jacobson, Michael F; and Maxwell, Bruce. *What Are We Feeding Our Kids?* Workman Publishing, 1994.

Jaffrey, Madhur. *Madhur Jaffrey's World-of-the-East Vegetarian Cookbook.* Alfred A. Knopf, 1987.

Klaper, Michael. *Pregnancy, Children, and the Vegan Diet.* Gentle World, 1988.

Kleinman, Ronald E., ed. *Pediatric Nutrition Handbook,* Fourth Edition. The Committee on Nutrition, American Academy of Pediatrics, 1998.

La Leche League. *The Womanly Art of Breast-feeding.* Penguin Putnam, 1997.

Langley, Gil. *Vegan Nutrition.* Vegan Society, 1995.

Lozowick, Lee. *Conscious Parenting.* Hohm Press, 1997.

Marcus, Erik. *Vegan: The New Ethics of Eating.* McBooks Press, 1998.

Melina, Vesanto; Davis, Brenda; and Harrison, Victoria. *Becoming Vegetarian: The Complete Guide to Adopting a Healthy Vegetarian Diet.* Book Publishing Company, 1995.

Messina, Mark; and Messina, Virginia. *The Dietitian's Guide to Vegetarian Diets: Issues and Applications.* Aspen Publishers, 1996.

Messina, Virginia; and Messina, Mark. *The Vegetarian Way: Total Health for You and Your Family.* Three Rivers Press, 1996.

Murray, Michael T.; and Butler, Jade. *Understanding Fats & Oils.* Progressive Health Publishing, 1996.

Reno, Liz; and Devrais, Joanna. *Allergy Free Eating: Key to the Future.* Celestial Arts, 1992.

Roehl, Evelyn. *Whole-food Facts: The Complete Reference Guide.* Healing Arts Press, 1996.

Shelov, Steven P.; and Hannemann, Robert E., ed. *Caring for Your Baby and Young Child: Birth to Age 5* (revised edition). The American Academy of Pediatrics, 1998.

Shurtleff, William; and Aoyagi, Akiko. T*he Book of Tofu: Protein Source of the Future—Now.* Celestial Arts, 1998.

Spock, Benjamin; and Parker, Steven J. *Dr. Spock's Baby and Child Care.* Simon & Schuster, 1998.

Tamaro, Janet. *So that's what they're for! Breast-feeding Basics.* Adams Media Corporation, 1998.

Tamborlane, William V., ed. *The Yale Guide to Children's Nutrition.* Yale University Press, 1997.

Yntema, Sharon. *Vegetarian Children.* McBooks Press, 1995.

_____.*Vegetarian Pregnancy.* McBooks Press, 1994.

The United States Department of Agriculture, Human Nutrition Information Service. *Agriculture Handbook Number 8: Composition of Foods Handbook.*

Reference Websites

Amazon.com   http://www.amazon.com

American Society for Nutritional Sciences: Nutrition Information
http://www.faseb.org/asns

Charles Attwood, M.D.   http://www.vegsource.org/attwood

The China-Cornell-Oxford Project
http://www.nutrition.cornell.edu/chinaproject

Compassionate Action for Animals   http://www.ca4a.org

Cornell University Division of Nutritional Sciences
http://www.human.cornell.edu/dns/DNShome.html

The Farm   http://www.thefarm.org

The International Childbirth Education Association, Inc.
http://www.icea.org

The International Lactation Consultant Association
http://www.erols.com/ilca

International Vegetarian Union   http://www.ivu.org/articles/stats.html

La Leche League International   http://www.lalecheleague.org

Loma Linda University and Medical Center   http://www.llu.edu

Michael Klaper, MD   http://www.vegsource.org/klaper

National Academy of Sciences   http://nationalacademies.org/

The Polynesian Voyaging Society   http://leahi.kcc.hawaii.edu/org/pvs/

Sci-Veg: Scientific Discussion of Vegetarian Issues
http://www.sci-veg.org

United States Food and Drug Administration   http://www.fda.gov

United States Department of Agriculture   http://www.usda.gov

Vegan.com   http://www.vegan.com

VegSource   http://www.vegsource.org

William Harris, M.D.   http://www.vegsource.org/harris

World Health Organization   http://www.who.int

Index

Pyridoxine. *See* Vitamin B-6

Questions, about diet, 116–117, 243
Quinoa, 168, 201, 213, 223

Raising Healthy Kids (Kushi), 37
Rastafarians, 55
Raw Foodist, definition of, 29
Raw foods, 36, 210
RDA (Recommended Dietary
    Allowances), 99
  guidelines for, 61, 62, 63
  for protein, 69
Recipes, 52, 176, 220–229
Recommended Daily Allowances
    (RDA), 62
Record-keeping, 117
Red Star Vegetarian Support Formula,
    78, 191–192
Rennin, 190
Reno, Liz, 239
Retinol Equivalents (RE), 73
Rhubarb, 202
Riboflavin. *See* Vitamin B-2
Rice, 168, 170, 213
Rice cereal, 200, 202, 213
Rice Pudding recipe, 228–229
Rickets, 55
Ripault, Chris, 145
Rise and Shine Quinoa Cereal recipe,
    223
Rye, 168–169

Salt. *See* Sodium
*San Francisco Bay Area Baby
    Resource Guide* (Belden), 115
Sanitation
  bottles and, 158–159
  eggs and, 188–189
  factory farming and, 96
  in India, 42
  organic foods and, 242
  vitamin B-12 and, 78
Saturated fats, 71
Say Sesame Milk recipe, 221
*Sea Vegetable Gourmet Cookbook and
    Wildcrafter's Guide, The*
    (Lewallen), 192–193
Sea vegetables, 192–193
Seasonal foods, 156

Seitan, 170
Selenium, 89
  RDA for, 99
Self-demand feeding, 197, 204–206
Semi-essential amino acids, 68
Serving sizes, 136, 208–209
Sesame seeds, 179
Seventh-Day Adventists, 26, 31–33
Shintani, Dr. Terry, 47
Silicon, 91
Snack suggestions, 217–219
Society, 54
Sodium, 44, 83–84
  calcium loss and, 80–81
  macrobiotic restrictions on, 35–36
Solid foods, introducing. *See* Weaning
Soups, 211
Soy beans, 172, 175, 203
Soy milk, 199, 203
Spelt, 169
Spinach, 202
Spock, Dr. Benjamin, 19, 167, 197, 198
Sprouts, 171–172, 174, 211
Squash, 202
Sunflower seeds, 179
Sunlight, 74, 234
Supplementary foods, 190–191
  list of, 191–193
Supplements, 97–98, 203, 234–235
  breast-feeding and, 64
  macrobiotic restrictions on, 36–37
Sustainable farming, 241–242
Sweet Orange Sweet Potatoes recipe,
    226–227
Sweet potatoes, 183, 201, 202
Sweeteners, 221

Taiwan, 38, 39
Tannins, 88
  protein absorption and, 69
Taster, child as, 184
Taurine, 68
Tea, herbal, 108
Teeth, 80, 86, 145, 237–238
Teff, 169
Thiamin. *See* Vitamin B-1
Tobacco smoke, calcium loss and, 81
Tofu, 124, 172, 203, 210, 223
Tomatoes, 183
Tooty-Fruity Salad recipe, 225–226

Trace minerals, 84–91
Trans-fatty acids, 71
Triticale, 169

Umbilical cord, clamping of, 87
Upper Intake Levels (UL), 63

Vanadium, 91
Veg*n, definition of, 27–28
Vegan
  allergies and, 199–200
  definition of, 27
  health of children and, 57
  protein and, 69
  serving guideline for, 135, 209
Vegetables
  introducing to diet, 202
  juices from, 211
  listed, 182–184
  in macrobiotic diet, 36
  overcoming dislike of, 231–233
  selection, storage, and handling of,
    180–181
  serving sizes for, 136, 208
Vegetarian Children (Yntema), 54, 237
Vegetarian, definition of, 27
Vegetarian Resource Group, 117
Vegetarian Society of Georgia, 125
Vegetarian Times, 176
Vitamin A, 72–73
  RDA for, 99, 133
Vitamin B-1 (Thiamin), 76
  DRI for, 100, 134
Vitamin B-2 (Riboflavin), 76
  DRI for, 100
Vitamin B-3 (Niacin), 76
  copper absorption and, 85
  DRI for, 100
Vitamin B-6 (Pyridoxine), 76
  DRI for, 100, 134
  in goats' milk, 77
Vitamin B-12 (Cobalamins), 56, 77–79
  deficiencies of, 55
  DRI for, 100, 134
  in macrobiotic diet, 37
  during pregnancy, 106
Vitamin C (Ascorbic acid), 40, 79
  copper absorption and, 85
  iron absorption and, 88
  RDA for, 99, 133

Vitamin D, 56, 73–74
  in breast milk, 64
  calcium absorption and, 80
  DRI for, 100, 134
  phosphorus and, 82
  during pregnancy, 106–107
Vitamin E, 74–75
  RDA for, 99, 133
Vitamin K, 75
  RDA for, 99, 133
Vitamin supplements, 234–235

Waianae Diet, 47
Walnuts, 179–180
Water, 84, 93–94, 110
Water-soluble vitamins, 76–79. *See
  also specific vitamins*
Weaning, 111–113, 144–146, 200–207
Weight gain, during pregnancy, 104
Weight loss, of child, 197, 204, 239
Wet-nurse, 195
Wheat, 169–170, 213
Wheat germ, 210
White, Ellen G., 31–32
White, Thelma, 48
Working Party, India, 51–53
World Health Organization, 49, 151

Yeast, nutritional, 191–192, 210
Yin and yang, 34
Yntema, Sharon
  on child development, 137
  on feeding schedules, 146
  on finding right foods, 154–155
  on natural development of child,
    243–244
  on nutrition guidelines, 61–62
  on other cultures, 25
  on pregnancy, 102
  on preparing foods, 113–114
  on raising vegetarian child, 118–122
  on vegetarianism, 21–24
  on weaning, 111
Yoga, 26
Yogurt, 163, 176, 190, 203, 210

Zen Macrobiotics (Ohsawa), 34
Zinc, 90
  during pregnancy, 108
  RDA for, 99, 133